HEALTH at GUNPOINT

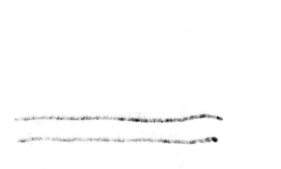

HEALTH at GUNPOINT

THE FDA'S SILENT WAR AGAINST HEALTH FREEDOM

JAMES J. GORMLEY

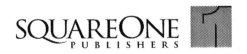

SQUAREONE
PUBLISHERS

Cover Designer: Jeannie Tudor
Cover Photo: SuperStock
Editor: Colleen Day
Typesetter: Gary A. Rosenberg

Square One Publishers
115 Herricks Road
Garden City Park, NY 11040
(516) 535-2010 • (877) 900-BOOK
www.squareonepublishers.com

Library of Congress Cataloging-in-Publication Data

Gormley, James J.
  Health at gunpoint : the FDA's silent war against health freedom / James J.
Gormley.
    pages cm
  Includes bibliographical references and index.
  ISBN 978-0-7570-0381-3 — ISBN 0-7570-0381-8
  1. United States. Food and Drug Administration. 2. Pharmaceutical
policy—United States—Evaluation. 3. Food adulteration and inspection—
United States—Evaluation. 4. Public health—United States—Evaluation. I. Title.
  RA401.A3G67 2013
  362.17'82--dc23
                              2013001139

ISBN 978-0-7570-0381-3

Printed in the United States of America

10   9   8   7   6   5   4   3   2   1

Contents

Acknowledgments

Thanks are first due to Frank Murray for his 1984 book, *More Than One Slingshot: How the Health-Food Industry Is Changing America,* as *Health At Gunpoint* is its successor, both in subject and in spirit.

A great deal of appreciation is also owed to all natural health pioneers and advocates of health freedom, past and present. I especially thank Clinton Ray Miller, James Turner, Beth Clay, Roy Upton, Bill Crawford, Chanchal Cabrera, Dana Ullman, Jonathan Emord, Alex Schauss, Iva Lloyd, Michael Stroka, and Scott Tips.

I feel deep gratitude to my wife, Juana, and our kids, Julian and Natalia, for putting up with—and encouraging—me and my penchant for poring over archival records and old books, even in the wee hours of the night!

Thanks go out as well to the wonderful team at Square One Publishers, especially Colleen Day, who is a consummate editor, a gifted writer, and a joy to work with.

A final word of appreciation is owed to you, dear reader. By choosing this book and empowering yourself with the information it contains, you have joined the illustrious ranks of all those who seek health justice and health freedom for future generations.

Of course, I also offer an apology for any errors of commission or omission—which are mine alone—in the hope that even an imperfect gem can shine brightly.

Foreword

I remember when James Gormley answered an ad in the *New York Times* for associate editor of what was then called *Better Nutrition for Today's Living* magazine at the beginning of 1995. I was curious to see if he would "get" the nutrition-for-optimal-health angle, since he had previously been an editor of medical journals. Little did he know that the article test I had given him—to do a thorough overview of Linus Pauling and vitamin C—was an especially tough test for any candidate, since I had a special interest in the topic and had written about it extensively. But James passed the test with flying colors, and I then knew that he had "right stuff" to join the magazine that I had shepherded for so many years.

After some months, when I moved on to run a health magazine group based in California, I knew that I was leaving the magazine in very capable hands, and that James would do well in the job of editor-in-chief of what is now known as *Better Nutrition* magazine. However, I could never have foreseen the great gusto and passion with which he would throw himself into the fray. Practically from day one, James was testifying in support of dietary supplement rights on Capitol Hill, leading grassroots health freedom campaigns, lecturing on organics and health, and even doing a great deal of radio and TV interviews, often going head-to-head with health food industry critics.

James well understood nutrition science and always led with his strongest suit. His arguments were unerringly based on science and supportive of the consumer's right to the best possible level of health, the finest high-potency products, and full access to information on those products and health-improving regimens. As the years went by, he would become an expert in dietary supplement regulation, traveling to China, Iceland, Paris, and Rome in support of consumer health and health freedom. In the late 1990s, when I suggested to James that he consider continuing the health freedom story that was begun in my 1984 book, *More Than One Slingshot: How the Health Food Industry Is Changing America*, he was very enthused about the idea, and never gave up the goal of penning an updated story and call-to-action.

We can always rely on James Gormley and other enthusiastic watchdogs to keep us informed about government hypocrisy and its attempts to erode our freedoms. Fortunately, there is an army of concerned citizens who agree with us. While I have castigated the Food and Drug Administration (FDA) for its belligerent attitude, I should point out that there are many hardworking rank-and-file employees at the agency who are passionate about the health of Americans.

In *Health at Gunpoint*, James Gormley has done a masterful job of not only telling the health freedom story and giving credit to many of the early pioneers, but also of shining a light on the FDA's disgraceful record. Better still, he provides an international backdrop of the health freedom struggle, and empowers today's generation of health freedom fighters, wherever they live, with knowledge and tactics that will be invaluable to them and all future generations of global consumers who cherish liberty and self-determination above all.

Frank Murray
Professional health writer and
author of *More Than One Slingshot*

Introduction

n the United States today, there is, perhaps, no greater source of controversy than the subjects of health and healthcare. A growing number of Americans are dissatisfied not only with the regulations and outrageous costs associated with healthcare, but also the inadequacy of many conventional medical treatments, as evidenced by the increasing popularity of alternative and complementary medicine. Unfortunately, over the last several decades, medical and government authorities, especially the Food and Drug Administration (FDA), have taken steps to restrict access to natural therapies and disseminate inaccurate information about natural products—all the while approving and promoting unsafe pharmaceuticals and food additives that put the nation's health at risk.

It is this essential conflict that gave rise to the health freedom movement, a loose coalition of natural health advocates who actively oppose measures taken by the FDA, industry lobbyists, and politicians that reduce health choices. The movement also seeks to make consumers more aware of the risks of using certain medications and eating certain foods, as well as the potential benefits of natural healing methods and remedies. *Health at Gunpoint* is part of this movement, and each chapter presents a distinct piece of the decades-long fight for health freedom.

Chapter One provides historical background on the U.S. natural health movement, which arose in the nineteenth century and was influenced by factors such as deadly mainstream medicine, urbanization, poverty, and "mini-movements" like temperance, right-living, and physical culture. Chapter Two then traces the development of U.S. agriculture, which has become increasingly controlled by big business and politics and, in turn, a source of nutritionally bankrupt crops that negatively affect both the food supply and environment. As you will see, the problems stemming from commercialized agriculture have spurred health food advocates and environmentalists alike to call for a return to natural and sustainable ways of producing and consuming food.

In Chapter Three, you will learn about the major political milestones that have determined and shaped policies towards dietary supplements and natural products. These battles, fought mainly between the FDA and the natural health industry, culminated in the passage of the Dietary Supplement Health and Education Act (DSHEA) of 1994, the law that governs rights regarding dietary supplements today. Many believe that this legislation is the sole legal document standing between consumer freedom in the United States and the more restrictive inclinations of the FDA.

The final two chapters consider natural health in the U.S. within a global context. Chapter Four focuses on the Codex Alimentarius Commission, or simply "Codex," an international body established in 1963 to set food purity standards and guidelines. While the stated purpose of Codex was to protect and serve the public health, it has become strongly influenced by the European Union, which is much more restrictive than the United States when it comes to dietary supplements. In other words, European regulations and Codex guidelines may soon hinder, rather than facilitate, health freedom by attempting to standardize and globalize food and food products.

Chapter Five, which is centered on the current situation in Canada, provides a glimpse at what may happen in the United States if globalization (euphemistically referred to as "harmonization") of international regulations is pursued. Due largely to the country's close cultural, social, and political ties to Europe, Canada is more prohibitive when it comes to supplements and yet more open-minded in its attitude towards traditional healing methods. Now at a crossroads in terms of health policy, "The Canada Example" reveals where the United States could be headed as well if consumers do not take action and demand more changes—and accountability—from Big Pharma, Big

Agriculture, the medical establishment, and government authorities like the FDA.

Health at Gunpoint was written not only to shed light on the troubling decisions that the FDA has made for over a century, but to prepare you, the consumer, for the present and future battles facing your health. The world in which we live is controlled by lobbyists and money, and it's crucial that you understand how these factors impact your well-being. By uncovering the silent war that has been waged on public health, you will be in a better position to preserve and safeguard your health rights and freedom.

1

The Origins of the U.S. Natural Health Movement

"We have been given the work of advancing health reform."

—ELLEN G. WHITE, A FOUNDER OF THE SEVENTH-DAY
ADVENTIST CHURCH, 1902

The natural health movement in the United States formed as a result of several forces and mini-movements that created a "perfect storm" of influence. The barbaric state of mainstream medicine during the nineteenth century played a role, as did widespread problems with public sanitation, food safety, and water purity. The emergence of health-oriented religious groups, which advocated nutrition, cleanliness, and temperance, also helped plant the seeds of health consciousness among the American public. In addition, traditional healing practices of Native Americans, as well as European practitioners of natural medicine gave way to a uniquely American model of naturopathy that would inspire people to seek alternative treatment over the widely available—and often toxic—remedies that were part of conventional medical practice. This chapter explores each of these forces, many of which occurred concurrently, and shows how they culminated not only in the formation of the natural health industry, but also in the first legal and political battles to preserve our health freedom.

AN INTRODUCTION TO NATURAL HEALTH IN THE U.S.

Despite the commonly held idea that the "old days" were more wholesome and pure in every way, old-time America was a hard-drinking,

5

poor-eating age saddled with deadly poisonous medicine, filth, child labor, contagious disease, poverty, malnutrition, and even starvation. Abominable conditions, both in mainstream medical practice and society in general, paved the way for health campaigners and right-living preachers to have a voice in America—and one that strongly resonated with the public. This section takes a look at various cultural forces at work in the U.S. during the mid-nineteenth century in order to make sense of the health- and medicine-based movements that would soon emerge.

Mainstream Medicine

The natural medicine and health movements were a reaction to the barbaric state of mainstream medicine in the late eighteenth and nineteenth centuries typified by such modalities as mercury-based "medicines" and bloodletting—a practice of withdrawing small amounts of blood in order to "cure" an illness. Such practices were certainly worse than any disease, usually to a fatal degree. Elisha Bartlett wrote the following in 1848 as a reaction to the horrific state of affairs in the conventional medicine of the time:

> [The] general confidence which has heretofore existed in the science and art of medicine . . . has within the last few years been violently shaken and disturbed, and is now greatly lessened and impaired. The hold with which medicine has so long had upon the popular mind is loosened; there is a widespread skepticism as to its power of curing diseases, and men are everywhere to be found who deny its pretensions as a science, and reject the benefits and blessings which it proffers them as an art.

According to Dana Ullman, a homeopathic expert, "There is general agreement among medical historians today that orthodox medicine of the 1700s and 1800s in particular frequently caused more harm than good." In addition to bloodletting and leeches, doctors also commonly used so-called *patent medicines*, concoctions that were promoted as cures containing rare and exotic ingredients but, in reality, consisted of toxic substances like arsenic, lead, laudanum (a tincture of opium), and mercury. Some, such as Whitehead's Essence of Mustard, were packed with a whopping percentage of hard liquor, ardent spirits, and even turpentine. Tragically, these nostrums—which were offered by mainstream doctors and peddlers alike—were often more dangerous than the conditions they were supposed to treat.

Mercury-laced patent medicines like Swaim's Panacea (see the inset below) were especially popular in the United States during this period. In fact, mercury—also referred to as calomel—was the second most popular purgative in conventional medicine of the nineteenth century and the second most popular drug after opium. Typical side effects of the substance included severe mouth ulcers, rotting of the jawbone, and fetid salivation. It was also known to cause patients' teeth to fall out.

According to Kelly Harmon in her 2003 dissertation on patent medicines, the use of patent medicines increased in the mid-nineteenth century for several reasons, including declining health among the U.S. population and a general distrust of traditional doctors. Westward expansion was also a factor, since people residing on the isolated frontier did not have access to real medical care. Low cost, availability, and increased advertising also played a role in the prevalence of patent remedies. The 1897 Sears Roebuck catalog, for

---

Swaim's Panacea

"The advertisements in our newspapers testify to the number and wonderful healing powers of the numerous vegetable syrups made and sold in this city [Philadelphia], under the title of Panacea.

In a report made by a committee of the Philadelphia Medical Society two years ago, on the subject of quack medicines, a number of instances are given of mercurial salivation, produced by taking Swaim's Panacea.

The public, with its ready credulity, will not perhaps consider this discovery of any moment: they have now only to believe the mercury, given by ignorant quacks, is a safe, mild, and uniformly efficacious thing; and that it is only to be feared when prescribed by a discerning and conscientious physician.

Surely this little additional stretch of faith, cannot be any great effort for those who have chosen to overlook all the rules of logic and common sense, in favour of a mercurialized syrup of sarsaparilla, yclep'd Swaim's Panacea."

—*The Journal of Health*, vol. 1, no. 6. November 25, 1829

example, offered several pages of patent medicines and elixirs for sale via mail order.

Furthermore, restrictions on alcohol—a result of the temperance movement—made alcohol-containing patent medicines popular among Civil War soldiers in particular, since alcohol rations to soldiers were strictly limited and heavily taxed. Since most Civil War fatalities (400,000 out of 620,000) were due to sickness and disease rather than actual combat, surviving soldiers became great advocates of patent medicines, claiming (however incorrectly) that they were the reason they were alive. Of course, it is clear that addiction to alcohol, as well as other ingredients like opium, morphine, and cocaine, also contributed to widespread popularity of patent medicines.

Nevertheless, Americans would begin to demand alternatives to the literally poisonous concoctions. Increased exposure to food contamination, pollution of the air and water, and the horrible state of sanitation—especially in cities—only added fuel to the reform fire.

Living Conditions in the Cities

Dangerous medical practice was not the only social condition that fueled the fires of health reform in the 1800s. As Ronald Numbers explained in his 1976 book, *Prophetess of Health: A Study of Ellen G. White:*

> For all its apparent vitality, America in the early nineteenth century was a sick and dirty nation. Public sanitation was grossly inadequate and personal hygiene virtually nonexistent. The great majority of Americans seldom, if ever, bathed. Their eating habits, including the consumption of gargantuan amounts of meat, were enough to keep most stomachs perpetually upset. Fruits and green and leafy vegetables seldom appeared on the table, and the food that did appear was often saturated with butter or lard.

Poor immigrants who settled in American cities during the mid-1800s and early 1900s typically lived in tenements rife with filth, disease, and crime. Tenement houses, such as those in New York City, also often lacked drainage and proper ventilation. According to Miriam Medina, immigrants were forced to "live in damp, smelly cellars or attics," with eight to ten men, women, and children packed into small single rooms. Her description of housing conditions paints an alarming picture of what immigrants endured:

> As you entered the overcrowded tenement buildings, you were greeted with a nauseating stench emanating from unwashed bodies, dirty rags, old bottles, stale cooking odors and accumulating garbage heaps in the rooms. Decaying grease adhering to waste pipes from kitchen sinks added its putrid odor to the foul emanations. These tenement buildings were dangerous firetraps, as well as a breeding place for murderous rodents that would kill babies in their cribs.

In cities, garbage and chamber-pot slop were thrown into the streets, "left to fester in the scorching sun. Along the streets, one would find in various stages of decomposition dead dogs, cats or rats," wrote Medina. Adding to the nightmarish scenario was the fact that child labor across the nation was rampant, with small children even working night shifts at toxin-spewing factories.

Despite the efforts of sanitarians to reduce urban filth (see the inset on page 10), these wretched conditions served as an ideal breeding-ground for disease. Cholera was especially rampant, hitting millions of people as it spread from northeastern India along trade routes in the late 1820s, and then across Europe in the early 1830s. According to the CUNY Graduate Center's Virtual New York website, "Cholera reached North America in June 1832, first appearing in Quebec, Canada, on June 6, and then traveling down the St. Lawrence to the Hudson River." In only two months, cholera killed approximately 3,500 New York City residents, the majority of whom were black or Irish and living in the slums. The disease, which was commonly treated with bloodletting, laudanum, and mercury, would eventually kill many thousands more due to subsequent outbreaks in 1839 and 1866.

With widespread disease, high infant mortality rates, horrible living conditions, and great numbers of factory deaths, life expectancy for men was only fifty-three years by the early 1900s. Women's life expectancy at fifty-four was only marginally better. By 1918, one in five American children did not survive beyond five years of age. In some cities, the situation was even worse, with 30 percent of infants dying before their first birthday. Childhood diseases such as diphtheria, measles, scarlet fever, and whooping cough contributed to these high death rates.

According to Elizabeth Fee in 1994's *The History of Public Health and the Modern State,* "The first expressions of concern for public health came not from the federal government, or even the states, but from the rapidly growing eastern cities." Each city tackled the problems of disease, squalor, and inhuman living conditions in its own ways. "Poverty and disease could no longer be treated simply as individual failings; they were becoming social and political problems of massive proportions," Fee added.

In fact, according to Nina E. Redman in *Food Safety* (2007), in the 1880s, women organized protests to demonstrate against vile work conditions in New York City slaughterhouses, for example, as well as against food contamination in many parts of the country. Thankfully, in the early 1900s, Upton Sinclair's *The Jungle* ushered in a new era of improved food production and working conditions. Around the same time, new visions of health developed in Europe and the U.S., such as naturopathy, clean living, and the physical culture movement, which often overlapped.

Healers, Health Campaigners, and Right-Living Advocates

Along with the push for better conditions in housing, sanitation, and medicine, there emerged a number of mainly religious leaders whose

Sanitarians and Disease

In the 1800s, most physicians and public health experts believed that disease was caused not by microorganisms but by dirt. Thus, sanitarians at the time believed that cleaning dirt-infested cities and building better sewage systems would prevent and put an end to many epidemics. Cities and towns across the country took steps to improve local sewage systems and make clean water more accessible to residents. These improvements led to a significant decline in gastrointestinal infections and mortality rates among infants, children, and young adults by 1918. However, since bacteria that reside in dirt is not the cause of every disease, this approach was not effective in ending all epidemics.

evangelizing focused on temperance (abstention from alcohol), cleanliness in the home, and a diet based on purity and simplicity. This is hardly surprising, given the fact that the United States during this time was a hard-drinking, poor-eating, and dirty place. A classic passage from the *Journal of Health* in 1829 says it all:

> If a plain and temperate diet, a due degree of appropriate exercise, pure air, proper clothing, in connexion with an unsullied conscience and a cheerful mind—were the remedies to which men were in the habit of resorting, to sustain the strength of their systems, the *'mens sana in corpore sano'* [sound mind in sound body] would be a far more common possession than is now the case.

The movements that embodied these ideas shared a distaste for heroic medicine—a term for dangerous mainstream medical practices such as bloodletting, surgery, and patent remedies—as well as a preference for vegetarianism. A few key movements are discussed in the pages that follow.

Shakers

Before the rise of naturopaths and health crusaders in nineteenth century, there was Ann Lee (1736–1784), the leader of the United Society of Believers in Christ's Second Coming, or the Shakers. In 1774, she and a small group of followers emigrated from England and settled in upstate New York. There they gained an enthusiastic following, with many claiming that Lee had spiritual gifts, including visions, prophecy, and special healing powers. Her touch was said to have "the power of God."

Lee, who was also a charismatic and riveting speaker, traveled around the colonies, especially the New England colonies, preaching her gospel views. Part of the Shaker message was also health-related. As adherents, they prohibited the consumption of pork, tea, and coffee. Interestingly, the group was the first to start the practice of selling seeds in paper packets, and they were one of the first mass producers of medicinal herbs in the United States. And although men were the ones to grow the crops in Shaker communities, it was the women who picked, sorted, and packaged the products to be sold. In other words, women were a valuable and indispensable asset in the community.

The Millerites and the Seventh Day Adventists

If there is one man that can be credited with starting the Seventh Day Adventist religious movement, it's William Miller (1782–1849), a former Baptist preacher who became an adherent of Deism, a school of thought using reason and the laws of nature to justify the existence of God. Miller developed the foundations of Adventist faith between 1815 and September 1822, when he published a twenty-point document focused on what he was convinced would be the imminent Second Coming of Christ. He began giving public lectures in 1831 and, in 1834, published a summary of his teachings entitled, *Evidence from Scripture and History of the Second Coming of Christ, about the Year 1844: Exhibited in a Course of Lectures.* He also met Ellen Gould Harmon in March 1840 on a trip to Portland, Maine, to warn residents of Christ's return. Harmon would later become a dedicated Millerite and reportedly experience several visions.

According to historian Ronald Numbers, the Millerite movement "exemplified the natural affinity between revivalism and temperance in nineteenth-century America." He also wrote that Miller, "who saw the hand of the Lord in the temperance societies springing up around the country, warned the expectant saints that those who drank [alcohol] would be 'wholly unprepared' for the Second Coming."

Although the Second Coming did not occur in 1844, as originally predicted by Miller and his followers, there were still very devout believers who carried the movement forward. In fact, it was in 1844 that Ellen experienced her first reported vision, in which she claimed to see "something of the travels of the Advent people to the Holy City [New Jerusalem]." Then, in 1846, she married James White, a young Millerite preacher who "never touched alcohol, tobacco, tea, or coffee, and a Cincinnati believer went even further by adding flesh foods [meat] to the list of forbidden articles." Two years later, Ellen White received the first of her many health-related visions. According to her estate, "Ellen [Harmon] White was given a vision of the relation of physical health to spirituality, of the importance of following right principles in diet and in the care of the body, and of the benefits of nature's remedies—clean air, sunshine, exercise, and pure water."

To a Seventh Day Adventist in the 1860s, health reform meant eating two meals per day consisting of fruits, vegetables, grains, and nuts. Following a vision of Ellen White in 1863, meat, eggs, butter, cheese, alcohol, coffee, and tea, were excluded from the diet. In her work *Ministry of Healing*, White also advocated "pure air, sunlight, abstemiousness, rest, exercise, proper diet, the use of water, trust in divine power—these are the true remedies."

Health Reformers and Campaigners

Perhaps no health reformer was more influential than Sylvester Graham (1794–1851). Best known today for his invention of what would later be called Graham Crackers, he was born in West Suffield, Connecticut in 1794—the seventeenth child of the seventy-two-year-old Reverend John Graham, Jr. Following in his father's footsteps, Graham decided to prepare for the ministry. He also studied languages at Amherst College for a short time in 1823. After enduring a protracted illness, he began preaching for the Presbyterian Church in New Jersey and, in 1830, was appointed as an official for the Pennsylvania Temperance Society.

It was likely out of concern for his own health that Graham became interested in human nutrition and physiology. He started giving lectures on these subjects and developed a vegetarian diet—the "Graham system"—that advocated the use of whole wheat bread, pure water, fresh fruits and vegetables, and "cheerfulness at meals." In addition to milling his own flour (Graham flour), Sylvester Graham also established boarding houses and succeeded in getting his lectures published. His most ambitious work, *Lectures on the Science of Human Life*, was published in 1839 and became a leading text on health reform. However, his popularity waned in 1840, and he died in 1851 before he could finish writing *The Philosophy of Sacred History*, a volume of lectures relating his theories on healthy living to Scripture.

According to Aaron Bobrow-Strain in his 2012 book, *White Bread: A Social History of the Store-Bought Loaf*:

Graham combined evangelical revival with scientific study of the body. Called 'Christian physiology' . . . this was not faith healing, but rather a conviction that all disease arose from a failure to conform one's bodily habits to the Laws of Nature, a scientific order designated by the Creator. . . . In an age when meals were gargantuan and greasy, vegetables brutalized by endless boiling, and constipation a national plague, Graham's dietary recommendations must have offered some relief to stuffed diners.

Of course, it is best to read Graham's own writings to fully understand his vision of health reform. In *Lectures on the Science of Human Life* (1839), Graham wrote:

But when I say that the simpler, plainer, and more natural the food of man is, the more perfectly his laws of constitution and relation are fulfilled, and the more healthy, vigorous, and long-lived will be his body, the more perfect his senses, and the more active and powerful may his intellectual and moral faculties be rendered by suitable cultivation. . . . By simple food I mean that which is not compounded and complicated by culinary process; by plain food I mean that which is not dressed with pungent stimulants, seasonings or condiments; and by natural food I mean that which the Creator has designed for man, and in such conditions as are a best adapted to the anatomical structure and physiological power of the human system.

The combination of dangerous mainstream medicine, food contamination, rampant disease, and the resulting emergence of health crusaders, created a cultural landscape that was ripe for a new approach to treating illness. Naturopathy, or natural medicine, would be a major influence in the formation of the more recent natural health movement.

THE EUROPEAN ROOTS OF NATURAL MEDICINE

The natural health movement in the U.S. was largely shaped by the naturopathic tradition in Europe, especially Germany, as well as the teachings of European pioneers of natural healing and natural foods. Over the past two decades, the United States has seen a slight resurgence of *naturopathy*, a medical art originating in Germany that uses natural elements like air, light, water, pure foods, and herbs to stimulate the body's own healing powers. This section takes a look at the some of the most influential figures who shaped Europe's tradition of holistic medicine.

Paracelsus (1493–1541)

While physicians of the sixteenth century thought that the human body was controlled exclusively by the stars and planets, Swiss-born Paracelsus was a believer in the healing power of nature in matters of human health. Well-acquainted with herbs and medicinal plants, Paracelsus was able to save the leg of a rich printer, Frobenius, from amputation by using his "knowledge of nature's inner healing power," said Siegfried Gursche, MH, a father of Canada's modern health food

Paracelsus' Influence on Natural Products Today

Paracelsus was among the first physicians who realized that the most important parts of a plant are not its leaves, bark, roots, or stems, but the substances that can be derived from these parts. He believed that plants help us the most when we can distill or extract their essence—what he referred to as "quintessence"— in the form of herbal tinctures. According to Joel L. Swerdlow, PhD, in *Nature's Medicine* (2000), Paracelsus' work "was a major step toward the present-day pharmaceutical approach toward plants: Isolate the pure form of plant constituents, particularly the active ingredient."

The natural products industry started focusing on "active ingredients" in the mid-1990s. This created some problems, however, as many supplements were incorrectly standardized—the process in which a certain ingredient in a product (usually the most beneficial) is concentrated in a set amount. The herbal supplement St. John's wort, for example, which is used to balance mood, was originally standardized to a percentage of hypericin and then later to a percentage of hyperforin.

More recently, some manufacturers have been hard at work developing full-spectrum botanical extracts, which more closely mirror what we find in the actual plant or herbal constituents. Today, we find extracts of all types, some standardized to certain levels of active ingredients, some billed as full-spectrum extracts, and some a combination of both. Regardless of the type, however, companies are increasingly using gentler approaches to extract plant ingredients. More natural solvents, as well as more sophisticated natural processing methods, are now being employed in order to produce the best herbal supplements possible.

industry. Eventually, Paracelsus became the official physician of Basel, Switzerland, and was offered a professorship at the University of Basel.

According to Kirchfeld and Boyle, Paracelsus often repeated the advice, "Mumia cures all wounds, protect them from external enemies and they will be healed." The "mumia" to which Paracelsus referred was "the inner balsam or life power inherent in all flesh." He rebelled against medieval practices that were considered mainstream medicine at the time, like dressing surgical wounds with cow manure, viper fat, moss, and feathers, instead insisting that wounds be kept clean. His continued criticism of these treatments led to his being exiled from the university and, as a result, almost a decade of poverty. With the publication of a major work in 1536, however, Paracelsus' reputation was restored, and he became sought after by noblemen and royalty.

That being said, according to Kirchfeld and Boyle, "All his praise of nature's healing power did not make Paracelsus a nature doctor," as he is credited with introducing chemical drugs like antimonial and arsenical compounds, lead nitrates, chlorides of iron and gold, copper sulphates, and bismuth and tin compounds. Nevertheless, Paracelsus is considered a pioneer in the field of natural health, as well as a major influence on the modern pharmaceutical approach to plants (see the inset on page 15).

Franz Mesmer (1734–1815)

During the late 1800s, *Mesmerism,* or magnetic therapy, experienced a brief wave of popularity. Invented by Austrian physician Franz Mesmer, magnetic therapy relied on hypnotism and the power of suggestion to help heal patients. The founder of Christian Science, Mary Baker Eddy, was greatly influenced by this system.

Among those most interested in this new method of healing was Theodosius Purland (1805–1881), an English surgeon and dentist who used Mesmerism for tooth extractions and surgeries. Purland insisted that Mesmerists were scientists, and that the medical community had failed to recognize the more than 300 cases in which Mesmerism had proven benefits, instead advocating anesthesia.

Samuel Hahnemann (1755–1843)

Homeopathy is an alternative form of medicine based on the idea that disease can be cured with small amounts of the same agents that caused it, or "like with like." This doctrine was developed by Samuel Hahnemann, a German physician who was highly critical of conventional medicine in Germany at the time, which included harmful so-called treatments like purgatives, bloodletting, and *emetics*, or vomit-inducing agents. He produced several papers on arsenic poisoning, dietetics, hygiene, and psychiatric care, compiling his results in a treatise entitled "Organon of rational therapeutics" and published in 1810. The sixth edition, published in 1921, is still used today as homeopathy's foundational text.

Hans Burch Gram is the doctor responsible for bringing homeopathy to America. Although he was born in Boston, Gram attended medical school in Europe, where he was introduced to homeopathy by a physician who had studied with Hahnemann. In 1825, he returned to the U.S. and settled in New York City, where he began to practice homeopathic medicine. At its peak in the late 1800s, there were 22 homeopathic medical schools in the United States and more than 100 homeopathic hospitals.

Although homeopathy declined in America in the mid-1900s, since the 1970s, it has experienced a resurgence. In fact, notes Ullman, "The rediscovery of homeopathy by the general public is even more encouraging. The magazine, *FDA Consumer* . . . reported a 1,000 percent increase in sales of homeopathic medicines from the late 1970s to the early 1980s."

Christoph Hufeland (1762–1836)

The German physician Christoph Hufeland is rarely credited with serving as a predecessor to the American naturopathic movement, despite being one of the most respected physicians of his time. In Germany, however, medical doctors who specialize in natural therapeutics revere him as what Kirchfeld and Boyle described as a "shining example of a truly holistic physician in the best Hippocratic tradition."

An early believer in the healing power of pure water, Hufeland had an open-minded approach to other therapies and modalities, such as homeopathy and Mesmerism (see pages 16 and 17). His strong interest in public health inspired him to have the first morgue built in Germany, which was in response to the terrifying problem of people being accidentally buried alive.

Hufeland is also known as the father of anti-aging, as he coined the term *macrobiotic*, a word for the art of prolonging life. George Oshawa (1893–1966), an admirer of Hufeland's work, borrowed the term *macrobiotics* to refer to the traditional grain-centered diet that he would later popularize in the 1950s and 1960s.

Vincent Priessnitz (1799–1852)

Born in a small village in southern Silesia (now the Czech Republic), Vincent Priessnitz is universally regarded as the "father of hydrotherapy," and some even consider him to be the very first true "nature doctor." Priessnitz was the first health practitioner who systematized a natural healing method based on pure water, fresh air, skin friction and kneading, a simple diet, fresh air, and exercise. His naturopathic method understood toxicity as an underlying cause of disease, chronic disease as a consequence of treating acute conditions with symptom-suppressive methods, and detoxification (healing crisis) as the basis for curing disease.

Like most nature doctors, Priessnitz was hounded by the authorities, who at one point raided and wrecked his home, convinced that he was using drugs or sorcery on his patients. According to Kirchfeld and Boyle in *Nature Doctors,* they even cut up his sponges. Of course, they found nothing.

Priessnitz is said to have treated over 40,000 patients, only 45 of whom died under his care. According to James C. Jackson, a naturopath who actually influenced Ellen Harmon White, "If Vincent Priessnitz had never done anything else for mankind but to have discovered and brought into use this form of hydrotherapy, he would have done enough to make himself immortal."

Father Sebastian Kneipp (1824–1897)

Few people would dispute the claim that Father Sebastian Kneipp is the most famous nature doctor of all time. Born in a small Bavarian town and ordained as a priest in 1852, he became known as the "cholera vicar" as early as 1854, a name he earned after successfully treating a number of people who had the disease. Although he is commonly associated with one area of hydropathy (see the inset on page 19), Kneipp was a strong proponent of a wider healing system based on five main

---

Hydrotherapy

Despite centuries of popularity in ancient Egypt, Greece, and Rome, *hydrotherapy,* also called *hydropathy,* seemed to fade into oblivion until it was rediscovered in the late eighteenth and early nineteenth centuries by Dr. J. S. Hahn (1696–1773), Professor E. F. C. Oertel (1764–1850), Vincent Priessnitz, and Father Sebastian Kneipp. Hydropathy reached the United States by the 1840s, and the first hydropathic facility opened in 1844. The proprietor of the facilities, David Campbell, also founded the *Water Cure Journal.*

---

principles: hydrotherapy (the medicinal use of water), herbalism, exercise, nutrition (a clean diet of whole grains, fruits, vegetables, and limited quantities of meat), and spirituality. One of his most significant contributions was his discovery that cold gushes of water directed to specific areas of the body could produce healing effects.

Kneipp was an enthusiastic follower of Priessnitz, and the two men have been compared in terms of their impact on the field of naturopathy. In his 1951 book, *Live Wisely—Live Well!*, Bernhard Detmar had this to say about these two pioneers of natural healing:

> Priessnitz practiced for about thirty years, Kneipp for about forty. Priessnitz treated altogether 40,000 patients, Kneipp many times that figure. Both men had great successes, and both were world-famous. . . . Both made fresh, cold water the basis of their treatment. Both . . . were inspired by love of their fellow-men and sympathy with those who suffered. Both were strong-minded personalities who rejected compromise. They are together the most outstanding representatives of natural healing methods so far.

Benedict Lust (1872–1945)

The person credited with bridging the schools of European and American naturopathy is Benedict Lust, a German immigrant who arrived in the United States in 1892.

Reportedly weakened by several operations and six vaccinations forced upon him in "different parts of the world," Lust developed a bad case of tuberculosis. Despite homeopathic and allopathic treatments, he wasted away and was expected to die.

This all changed when he returned to Germany to seek treatment from Father Kneipp. According to Kirchfeld and Boyle, after he started Kneipp therapy, "Lust's health began to improve, and in eight months he had completely regained his health." His return to the U.S. as Kneipp's official representative in 1896 marked the beginning of naturopathy in the United States, and he was eventually able to establish a Kneipp school, clinic, and magazine. Since many Americans were not familiar with Kneipp, however, Lust changed the name of his magazine from *Kneipp Water Cure Monthly* to *The Naturopath*. By 1898, Lust was directing a naturopathic sanatorium and health resort with "scores of faithful patients," as well as a popular Kneipp health food store.

In 1900, Lust founded the Yungborn Health Resort on sixty-five acres of land in Butler, New Jersey, which featured lectures, locally grown vegetarian food, hiking, swimming, yoga, group exercises and sun-bathing. He also purchased the rights to the name "naturopathy" from one of his followers, Dr. John Scheel, who had coined the term in 1895. Soon after, he founded the American School of Naturopathy, the first naturopathic medical school in the world, and established the American Naturopathic Association, the first national professional organization for naturopathic physicians. Following World War I, he published the *Universal Naturopathic Encyclopedia* for drugless therapy and *Nature's Path* magazine, a very progressive and inclusive publication that featured articles on Ayurveda and yoga, and introduced Americans to the teachings of esteemed Indian yogi Paramahansa Yogananda (1893–1952).

Lust's success and notoriety would not go unchallenged, however, as he faced several years of persecution from adherents of mainstream medicine, including the New York County Medical Association. He was arrested sixteen times by New York authorities and three times by federal authorities. The witch hunt against him waned after the Medical Association lost a libel case against Lust in the early 1900s.

Lust was certainly far ahead of his time in many ways, not only in how he utilized many different modalities and healing systems, but also in his views regarding allopathic medicine, which he wrote about in the *Naturopath and Herald of Health* in 1935:

The medical machine in this country is the greatest curse ever visited on America. It is interested in keeping the people sick by undermining their health by vaccination and other medical superstitions and crimes. Eventually the plans of the medical trust will cause widespread damage to the American people if they are not checked.

All in all, the European naturopathic tradition was immensely important to the art of natural healing in North America. More specifically, it inspired American healing systems, many of which integrated or explored aspects of European naturopathy, homeopathy, and even Mesmerism.

THE RISE OF NATURAL MEDICINE IN THE UNITED STATES

In addition to the influence of European naturopathy, natural medicine in the United States was also shaped by the botanical and traditional knowledge of Native Americans. This marriage of indigenous and European traditions resulted in movements that were uniquely American, like Thomsonianism, Eclecticism, chiropractic, and others.

Thomsonianism

Along with Native American traditional medicine, *Thomsonianism* is considered the first "alternative" medical system to be founded in the United States. The movement was developed in the 1790s by Samuel Thomson (1769–1843), a New Hampshire farmer and herbalist who believed that restoring the body's normal heat was the only way to cure disease. This involved steam baths, as well as combinations of plant extracts and other substances, such as lobelia (an emetic) and cayenne pepper extracts, that either heated the body or caused evacuation. Opening the paths of elimination, part of what we call detoxification today, was not unique to Thomsonianism; as you may recall, calomel was commonly offered by physicians and peddlers to induce vomiting and purgation.

Thomson sold patents, which he called "Family Rights," to families who wanted to use his system of medicine for twenty dollars. Right-holders who were enrolled in Thomson's Friendly Botanic Society were able to purchase Thomson's herbs and formulas, which he distributed from a central warehouse, along with a sixteen-page instruction booklet entitled, "Family Botanic Medicine." Thomson's method attracted large numbers of followers, as it was far less toxic than mainstream medicine at the time. After practicing for about ten years, Thomson expanded his booklet into a book called *New Guide to Health; or Botanic Family Physician* in 1822, which underwent several reprintings.

During the 1820s and 1830s, Thomsonian sales agents could be found throughout New England, as well as the southern and western United States, encouraging Americans to become their own doctors. This message resonated, and by 1840, Thomson had sold over 100,000 patents. By his own estimates, some 3 million people adopted his system during his lifetime. According to Berman and Flannery, the then contemporary physician and writer Daniel Drake observed that the devotees of Thomsonianism were not "limited to the vulgar. . . . Respectable and intelligent mechaniks, legislative and judicial officers, both state and federal barristers, ladies, ministers of the gospel, and even some of the medical profession 'who hold the eel of science by the tail' have become its converts."

Thomson took legal measures to protect his patented cures, which ensured others would not be able to make or sell lobelia pills. This "monopoly" was broken by Alva Curtis, a naturopathic physician who began teaching Thomson's system out of his home in 1835. He also created the so-called Independent Thomsonian Medical Society in 1835 to train practitioners, giving rise to the Eclectic movement.

Eclectic Medicine

The term "Eclectic medicine" was coined by Constantine Rafinesque (1784–1841), a physician who lived among Native Americans and learned their use of medicinal plants. Rafinesque applied the word "eclectic" to the use of any natural substance or method that was found to have health benefits. An extension of Thomsonianism and early American herbal traditions, Eclectic medicine was a reaction to the bloodletting and use of mercury-based remedies that were popular in the early nineteenth century. The Reformed Medical College was established by a medical tradesman, Wooster Beach, in 1829 in order to practice and teach Eclectic medicine. Drawing from therapies selected from both allopathic (conventional) and alternative schools of practice, Eclectic medical colleges sprang up and thrived. While they made use of many Thomsonian principles, Eclectic doctors were also trained in physiology and more conventional principles, along with botanical medicine.

The field expanded during the 1840s as part of a large populist movement in North America, and finally peaked in the 1880s and 1890s. In fact, by 1900, 20 percent of all doctors were what we call alternative physicians today; there were 10,000 homeopaths, 5,000 Eclectics, 5,000 other holistic doctors, and 100,000 allopaths. The schools that trained these non-traditional doctors were not approved by the infamous Flexner Report of 1910 (see the inset on page 24), which aimed to monopolize accreditation of medical schools in order to drive out non-allopathic medicine. By World War I, states and provinces were adopting curriculum requirements that closely followed those of the American Medical Association (AMA). This effectively forced Eclectic medical schools to either adopt the new model or shut down. Sadly, the last Eclectic medical school closed in Cincinnati in 1939.

Osteopathy

Osteopathy, originally a healing system based on musculoskeletal manipulation, was begun by Andrew Taylor Still (1828–1917) in the 1870s. Still was a doctor and army surgeon during the Civil War, a state and territorial legislator in Kansas, and one of the founders of Baker University. After years of practice and clinical observation, Still "concluded that what was called health care was mostly fixated on disease and that medicine per se consisted of the suppression of symptoms and little else," wrote Wayne Jonas, MD, and Jeffrey Levin, PhD, in *Essentials of Complementary and Alternative Medicine.*

Still developed the practice of osteopathy in Baldwin City, Kansas, where he lived during the Civil War. He named his new school of medicine "osteopathy" with the belief that "the bone, osteon, was the starting point from which [he] was to ascertain the cause of pathological conditions." In May 1892, Still founded the American School of Osteopathy, which is today called the A.T. Still University of the Health Sciences, in Kirksville, Missouri. Although the state of Missouri granted the school the right to award medical degrees, Still remained dissatisfied with conventional medicine and decided that his school would retain the distinction of the Doctor of Osteopathy (DO) degree.

Chiropractic Medicine

Chiropractic medicine was founded in 1895 by Daniel David Palmer (1845–1913) in Davenport, Iowa. Palmer, a magnetic healer, was convinced that manual manipulation of the spine could cure disease. His

---

The War Against
Naturopathic Doctors and Healers

In the mid-to-late nineteenth century, so-called conventional doctors and pharmacists were getting nervous. Medical herbalist Chancal Cabrera tells it this way:

> The "regular" doctors, as the [allopathic] medical practitioners were then called, were appalled at the success and popularity of the "irregulars" or herbal healers, most especially the Thomsonians. In 1847 the [AMA] was founded and it served as a focal point for the concerted effort to wipe out natural remedies in favor of the new drug remedies that were increasingly available. One way to do this was [to] issue licenses to practice medicine based upon achieving certain standards of competence. At the turn of the century the AMA initiated a study of the medical education establishments then available, including the herbal and Eclectic schools. Their requirements for approval included laboratories and texts that were not used or needed by the herbalists. When the AMA ran out of funding, the Carnegie Foundation stepped in and appointed Abraham Flexner to complete the study. The Flexner Report was released in 1910 and it was devastating to the herbal and Eclectic community. Within the next four years 29 schools closed down because they were not approved by the AMA, even though no-one in the AMA was actually qualified to properly assess the medicine they were teaching. Herbal and Eclectic medicine in the U.S. virtually died out for the next 60 years, preserved only in folk tradition and by Native Americans.

The mainstream pharmacies and the AMA joined together, after the Flexner Report of 1910, to almost completely close down the "competition" posed by the Eclectic, naturopathic, and homeopathic systems of medicine. By 1930, aside from osteopathic and chiropractic schools, alternative medicine had been dealt a severe blow.

---

first chiropractic patient was Harvey Lillard, who claimed that he had suffered from severely impaired hearing for approximately seventeen years, ever since he had experienced a "pop" in his spine. A few days after a spinal adjustment from Palmer, Lillard reported that his hearing was almost fully restored. Although he initially kept chiropractic a family secret, Palmer began teaching it to a few students at his new Palmer School of Chiropractic in 1898. One student, his son Bartlett Joshua Palmer, became an enthusiastic advocate of chiropractic and took over the school in 1906. Under his leadership, enrollment significantly increased.

Chiropractic competed with its predecessor osteopathy, which was also based on bone-setting, magnetic healing, and the idea that musculoskeletal manipulation improved health. Early practitioners of chiropractic believed that human beings had an innate life-force that represented God's presence within them, and that disruptions in this vital energy caused disease. Both Palmers considered declaring chiropractic a religion, which could have provided them with legal protection. Ultimately, however, they decided against it in order to avoid being confused with the Christian Science movement. Early chiropractors tapped into the populist movement as well, stressing the importance of hard work and industry, as well as allying themselves with the "common man" against the mainstream medical community.

THE PHYSICAL CULTURE MOVEMENT

Modern-day interest in the aesthetic development of the body, or physical culture, can be traced back to the Italian Renaissance, as demonstrated by the anatomically naturalistic masterpieces of Leonardo da Vinci and Michelangelo. Hundreds of years later, in the eighteenth and nineteenth centuries, an emphasis on youth fitness, especially for men, became a central message of nationalistic movements in Germany, France, Prussia, Sweden, Czechoslovakia, Poland, and Great Britain.

The physical culture movement in the United States came together as a result of several factors. The Industrial Revolution had created a new generation of workers who were office-bound and, therefore, sedentary—a problem made worse by the increasing use of cars. Adding to concerns was the rising ubiquity of processed foods that were low in cost but high in sugar and fat. In response, gymnasiums and schools, especially military academies, began to promote physical culture programs, which drew from such influences as folk games, military training, dances, sports, and calisthenics. There was also a new abundance of magazines and books focusing on exercise regimens and equipment. What today is known as the "Muscular Christianity" movement also played a role in advancing physical culture in the U.S. The movement emerged in the Victorian era and emphasized the connection between piety, physical well-being, and masculinity. Its first tangible manifestations in the United States were the creation of the Young Men's Christian Association (YMCA) and the pro-fitness preaching of world-famous evangelists like Dwight L. Moody.

Later, the physical culture movement would be spurred on by the belief that, as a matter of national pride, young people should be both fit and battle-ready. Ultimately, physical culture in the U.S. was a conglomerate of all of these factors, and emerged as a powerful evangelizing force in health reform. Some of the most influential figures and leaders of the movement are highlighted in the pages that follow.

Diocletian Lewis (1823–1886)

A strong argument can be made that the first American fitness guru was Diocletian Lewis, who, in addition to being a fitness advocate, was also a temperance campaigner, homeopath, and inventor of the beanbag. With his European-influenced system of calisthenics—exercises using one's own body weight rather than equipment—Lewis "was among the first to outline a program for improving one's life through exercise, a revolutionary idea at a time when complete rest was the preferred cure for stress-related symptoms and women, in particular, were often confined to bed and spoon-fed milk," wrote Mark Adams in his 2009 book, *Mr. America.* His drills were focused on improving hand-eye coordination, flexibility, and physical grace, and included lifting light weights, tossing beanbags, and swinging Indian clubs. In 1862, Lewis described his methods in his book, *The New Gymnastics for Men, Women and Children,* which became a bestseller.

George Windship (1834–1876)

Nicknamed "The Roxbury Hercules" and the "American Samson,"

George Windship was not just another promoter of light exercise, moderation, and vegetarianism. According to Jan Todd, PhD, of the University of Texas, "Windship's message was diametrically different. The body should be made as strong as possible, he contended, with no weak points." He developed a forty-minute daily strength-building routine, invented an adjustable dumbbell, and opened his own chain of gyms in the Boston area. His interest in heavy training went beyond the need or desire for muscle growth; he believed that heavy lifting was a highly effective form of medical therapy. This is the conviction behind his motto, "Strength is health."

He died of a massive stroke at the age of forty-two on September 12, 1876, which shed a negative light on heavy lifting as exercise. According to Dennis Mitchell of the United States All-Round Weight-lifting Association, "There were those who were against heavy lifting stating that it was dangerous, and used Dr. Windship's death as proof. It did have a negative affect on lifting, and for some years lifting was looked on as being dangerous."

Dudley Allen Sargent (1849–1924)

Dudley Allen Sargent directed both Harvard's Hemenway Gymnasium and the Normal School of Physical Training, which was later dubbed the Sargent School of Physical Education. An inventor of gymnasium equipment and the Sargent Anthropometric Chart, which tracked physical development, Sargent's work served to legitimize "physical culture as a teaching discipline under a new name, 'physical education,'" wrote Adams in *Mr. America.* His contributions to the discipline "spurred the idea that exercise and sports built character, which in turn fueled the astronomical growth of school sports."

William Blaikie (1843–1904) and Bernarr Macfadden (1868–1955)

A protégé of Sargent, William Blaikie was a strongman and endurance athlete, as well as an attorney and judge. He is also known for walking from Boston to New York—a total of 225 miles—in only four and a half days. His 1879 bestseller, *How to Get Strong and How to Stay So,* in which he presented a variety of Sargent-inspired exercises, served as an indictment of America's unfit youth and sedentary office workers.

In 1883, a copy of the book made its way into the hands of Bernard McFadden, the future physical culture icon who would be known as Bernarr Macfadden. According to Adams in *Mr. America*, "A friend would later compare the physical culturist's [Macfadden's] initial exposure [to Blaikie] to the day Thomas Carlyle cracked open one of Plato's works: 'He felt as if he were reading his own ideas, set down cogently and clearly, for the first time.'" Ben Yagoda wrote in a 1981 edition of *American Heritage* magazine that Macfadden was passionate about "the titanic benefits of exercise, the right foods, and periodic fasts, and the extreme perils of among other things, corsets, white bread, doctors, vaccination, overeating, and prudery. His public activities usually served to promote these ideas." In 1899, he founded the magazine *Physical Culture* and, twelve years later, published the five-volume *Encyclopedia of Physical Culture*, which totaled 2,969 pages. He also produced a wide range of books and pamphlets.

In 1905, Macfadden hosted the first big "physique contest" in the U.S., which continued to be held in New York City through the 1920s. According to Ben Yagoda, he also opened a chain of "one-cent Physical Culture restaurants—with menus strikingly similar to those of today's bean-sprout emporiums." Macfadden opened a number of spas as well, which he called "healthatoriums," in Chicago, Michigan, upstate New York, Long Island, and New Jersey's Pine Barrens, which he unsuccessfully tried to have incorporated as "Physical Culture City."

Many famous figures endorsed Macfadden's programs, including Henry Ford, George Bernard Shaw, and Upton Sinclair, who claimed that Macfadden taught him, free-of-charge, "more about the true principles of keeping well and fit for my work, than all the orthodox and ordained physicians, who charged thousands of dollars for it."

Unfortunately, Macfadden's campaign against prudery caused problems for him. His series of explicit articles on the dangers of syphilis, which were published in *Physical Culture*, resulted in a $2,000 fine. According to Yagoda, "only a pardon from President Taft saved him from a two-year prison term."

He rebounded in 1919 by launching *True Story,* a confession magazine that turned into a publishing empire. In fact, by the late 1920s, publications like *True Detective, True Story, True Romances, SPORT,* and the ever-popular *Photoplay* had reportedly netted Macfadden a fortune of $30 million. By 1935, the combined circulation of his magazines was 7,355,000, which was more than that of publishing giants like Hearst, Luce, and Curtis.

Charles Atlas (1892–1972)

Born Angelo Siciliano, Charles Atlas won two consecutive "Most Perfectly Developed Man" contests (created by Bernarr Macfadden) at Madison Square Garden in 1921 and 1922. He also performed a strong man act at the Coney Island Circus. According to the story Atlas often told, when he was a scrawny, 97-pound adolescent, a bully had kicked sand into his face at a beach. Determined to never repeat this humiliating experience, Atlas joined the YMCA and began a body-building regimen. In 1929, he founded Charles Atlas Ltd., which continues to market a fitness program for the "97-pound weakling."

Jack LaLanne (1914–2011)

Francois Henri "Jack" LaLanne, a famous exercise and nutrition expert and motivational speaker, has often been referred to as "the godfather of fitness" and the "first fitness superhero." When he was fifteen years old, LaLanne was said to have heard Paul Bragg, a health food advocate, give a lecture in which he discussed the "evils of meat and sugar." The talk inspired LaLanne, who likened the experience to being "born again."

In 1936, LaLanne opened what is considered to be the nation's first health and fitness club in Oakland, California. Here, he supervised exercise and offered nutritional advice with the goal of motivating people to improve their health. He later earned a Doctor of Chiropractic degree from the Oakland Chiropractic College and started the longest-running television exercise program, which first aired in 1951 and ran for thirty-four years. According to Joe and Ben Weider, the program was groundbreaking in that it spread "the message about healthy living and exercise decades before such things were generally accepted."

As writer Sam McManis wrote in a 2003 issue of *The San Francisco Chronicle*, LaLanne believed that processed foods were the reason for many health problems, as he noted that "a stream of aches and pains seems to encompass us as we get older." In his book *Revitalize Your Life*, which was published in 2003, LaLanne referred to the human bloodstream as a "River of Life" which is "polluted" by junk foods loaded with salt, sugar, preservatives, and artificial flavorings. In order to deal with disease and other ailments, LaLanne promoted a mostly meatless diet that included fish, as well as daily vitamin supplements.

The focus on physical culture often went hand-in-hand with an emphasis on healthy eating. Around the same time that LaLanne opened his first health and fitness club, leaders of the burgeoning health food movement gathered in Chicago to establish the industry's first trade association. A desire for pure foods and proper nutrition resulted in the birth of a movement that would directly lead to the natural health industry as we know it today.

HEALTH FOOD STORES EMERGE

In the groundbreaking 1984 book, *More Than One Slingshot: How the Health Food Industry is Changing America*, Frank Murray wrote that "a horrendous rape of the American food supply" started in the 1890s, when "millers purchased more sophisticated refining machinery [that] removed the germ, and many vitamins and minerals from wheat and other whole grains, and produced glistening, nutritionally inadequate white flour." This ravaging of the food supply did not go unnoticed. Between 1896 and 1938, the first health food stores opened in the U.S. In 1936, a Chicago baker named Anthony Berhalter organized a group of retailers and suppliers—or as they called themselves, "independent health food dealers"—who met in the Windy City and formed the American Health Foods Association (AHFA).

The first AHFA convention, which was held in 1937 at Chicago's Auditorium Hotel, consisted of fifteen booths and included early pioneering companies in the industry, such as Tam Products (today called American Health), Elam Mills, Battle Creek Scientific Foods, H.W. Walker, Inc., and Modern Diet Products. In 1938, the organization renamed themselves the National Health Foods Association (NHFA), whose first officers included such leaders in the field as Paul Bragg and Lelord Kordel (see the inset on page 33). The newly named association's first convention was held at Chicago's Sherman Hotel in the same year.

In these early days of health food stores, retailers did not offer an extensive line of products. As Stanley N. Phillipps, who ran Parks-Phillipps Special Foods in Ohio, told Murray in *More Than One Sling-*

shot, "Before the 1930s, there were very few health products to sell, except what we made or packaged, namely cracked wheat cereal, whole-wheat flour, 100% whole-wheat bread, Boston brown bread, unsulphured molasses, pure honey and sundried, unsulphured fruits, dates, raisins, prunes and figs." He added, "I learned that we could buy the famous Battle Creek Sanatorium Foods, and sell them, so we got the entire line of about 25 products." Products advertised in *Health Foods Retailing* magazine in 1938 include Alvita dehydrated tea, Bragg Meal Wheat Germ, the Fletcherizer blender, Franklin Mills flour, Hain Pure Foods, Henkle soy bean flours, Joyana soy bean drink (Tam Products), the Juicex Juicer (Hauser's Modern Diet Products), Kal vitamins, Parkelp kelp supplement, Pep-Ups (Energy Foods), San-O-Ban coffee substitute (Battle Creek Scientific Foods), and Swiss Kriss herbal laxatives (Hauser's Modern Diet Products).

During this time, the health food industry was characterized by a wonderful, supportive atmosphere. Health advocates ran ads in the only retail magazine *Health Foods Retailing*, for which they also wrote articles that further cemented their credibility and authority among health food dealers. They also gave talks around the country, which drew consumers to health food stores in those cities looking for the products endorsed by the speakers. As Stanley Phillipps told Frank Murray, his store's "first big boost came in 1932, when Paul Bragg came to town to open a big six-week program of lecturing and selling health products." Bragg, an engaging salesman and speaker, "packed the largest auditoriums in Cincinnati night after night, and when he left town we became the headquarters for all the products he recommended, and there was quite a line of them." In addition, Phillips said that "Gayelord Hauser was among the first very fine lecturers and, in his dignified way, he did a tremendous amount of educational work. . . . He was one of the most sought-after lecturers who ever came to Cincinnati." The most significant boon to health food stores in the early days, though, was books, especially ones written by Adelle Davis (see the inset on page 32), which brought scores of customers to health food stores in search of vitamins and other natural supplements.

Although the health food industry struggled throughout the war years, it regained its strength over a twenty-year period following World War II. In 1969, the NHFA merged with the American Dietary

Retailers Association and became the National Nutritional Foods Association (NNFA). The industry, now strengthened and united, was empowered in its ongoing battle against the Food and Drug Administration (FDA), which had started in 1966 when the agency imposed onerous and illogical restrictions on natural products. The industry scored important victories with the passage of the 1976 Vitamin Bill, and many years later, the Dietary Supplement Health and Education Act (DSHEA) of 1994. (See page 79 in Chapter 3). These laws, along with the more recent grassroots pro-natural health campaign, have forced the FDA to rethink its approach to regulating natural products and ingredients.

THE NATURAL HEALTH INDUSTRY SINCE 1994

Signed into law in 1994, the Dietary Supplement Health and Education Act (DSHEA) finally provided appropriate access to dietary sup-

---

The Great Health Food Pioneers of the Twentieth Century

Benjamin Gayelord Hauser (1895–1984). A German-American nutritionist and author, Hauser was reportedly cured of tuberculosis by Benedict Lust (see page 19), as well as a strict diet and herbal remedies provided to him by Brother Maier, a Swiss monk. Hauser later became a proponent of foods rich in vitamin B, while discouraging intake of sugar and white flour. His five so-called "wonder foods" were yogurt, brewer's yeast, powdered skim milk, wheat germ, and blackstrap molasses. In 1925, he joined the Milwaukee firm Modern Products, the manufacturer of Swiss Kriss, an herbal laxative developed by Hauser's brother-in-law, Sebastian Gysin. In 1927, he moved to Hollywood, where he became a successful author, lecturer, and nutritional advisor for celebrities. His most famous book was *Look Younger; Live Longer.*

Adelle Davis, MS (1904–1974). A leader in the field of holistic health, Davis was widely regarded as one of America's leading nutritionists. She worked as a private consulting nutritionist in California from 1931 to 1958, gaining popularity in the 1960s and 1970s due to public praise from *The New York Times, Life,* and the Associated Press. Her frequent appearances on *The Tonight Show*

---

plements. As sales exploded into a rarified zone of success that lasted well through 1997, the natural products (including health foods) industry appeared to be an unstoppable force. At the time, the biggest competitors for health food retailers were "kissing cousins" like Whole Foods, Wild Oats, and GNC, and many of the largest food and supplement manufacturers were still family-owned. In sum, the independent health food store reigned supreme. Then the bottom fell out.

Some of the biggest health food companies sold to pharmaceutical companies or went public with IPOs. Others acquired other companies in a wild frenzy of consolidation, or left the fold by trying mass-market distribution in order to increase their profits. Some of the companies that "jumped ship" would later try to return, with varying degrees of acceptance. Mass-market companies, such as Wal-Mart and big drug-store chains, bought out health food and supplement lines. Suddenly,

---

made Davis a celebrity and one of the most influential nutritionists in the United States. By 1974, her books had sold over 11 million copies since the publication of her first book, *Optimum Health*, in 1935.

Lelord Kordel, PhD (1904–2001). Kordel, a Polish-American nutritionist, supported the war effort during World War II by holding nutrition seminars and contributing to the "Food and Nutrition for Victory" programs, wartime talks that emphasized the importance of being fit and healthy for a stronger America. Following the war, Kordel authored several books, including *Health the Easy Way* (1946), *Health Through Nutrition* (1950), *Eat and Grow Younger* (1952), *Eat Your Troubles Away* (1955), *Cook Right—Live Longer* (1962), *Natural Folk Remedies* (1972), and *Eat and Grow Slender* (1977).

Carlton Fredericks, PhD (1910–1987). In 1957, Dr. Fredericks became a well-known voice in the United States with his radio program, "Design for Living," in which he took calls and gave nutritional advice. Specifically, he emphasized the importance of vitamin and mineral supplements, informing listeners that modern processing methods stripped foods of valuable nutrients. Although his advice was controversial at times, Dr. Fredericks was widely considered to be an expert in public health.

the health food industry became a much more unpredictable and volatile place in which to grow, thrive, and even survive.

Reflecting on the natural health marketplace as it exists today, Frank Murray said:

> After many years of being ridiculed by 'The Establishment,' the concepts of the health food industry are finally being legitimized— in that what it was saying 30 or 40 years ago is proving to be true. There are almost daily reports in the media on the value of vitamin C, calcium, vitamin E, fiber, vitamin D, folic acid and the other B vitamins, omega-3 fatty acids, etc. . . . The Establishment has painted itself into a corner, and it's reluctantly admitting that perhaps the health food industry was often right.

When asked about how he sees the marketplace now, Max Huberman (1934–2008), whose career and impact in the industry spanned several decades, replied, "My wife, Ruth, and I have always tried to stick to the principles of peace, justice and compassion, which are the same principles at the nucleus of the health food industry, with all of its contradictions." And when John R. Carlson (1934–2011), founder of Illinois-based Carlson Laboratories, was asked if the industry still has a soul, without missing a beat, he replied, "Yes. There are people out there who are very dedicated, people who care about improving the health of others more than they do about making money."

CONCLUSION:
THE FUTURE OF THE NATURAL HEALTH INDUSTRY

It's clear that the industry is evolving. Although imperfect, the natural health industry continues to be an oasis in a society and food industry dominated by processed, artificial, and often contaminated products. Max Huberman believed that consumers wanted "the real McCoy," meaning foods that are humanely produced, minimally processed, and free of GMOs and chemical additives. Commenting on the food sold in most supermarkets and restaurants today, Huberman said, "There's something wrong when we realize that people are walking around with full stomachs and they're starving to death," said Huberman. "In a typical 100 dollar supermarket wagon filled with groceries there isn't 100 cents worth of nutrition."

In 1939, John Maxwell, the Natural Product Association's first president, wrote the following advice for retailers in *Health Foods Retailing* magazine, words which ring as true today as they did sixty-five years ago:

> Watch the quality of the goods you sell. Give honest value in well-prepared foods, undenatured honest-to-goodness victuals. Stay clear of anything questionable and that cannot be proved to have merit as a real food. Set an ace-high standard. Give good, courteous and prompt service and your business should grow and endure. . . . Thus health food dealers will hold much of the future trade in their own hands; it will not drift away into other channels. Our places must be known as pure food emporiums if we are to have a good future.

2

Harvest of Shame
Business, Politics, and the Food Supply

"But when I say that the simpler, plainer, and more natural the food of man is, the more perfectly his laws of constitution and relation are fulfilled, and the more healthy, vigorous, and long-lived will be his body."

—SYLVESTER GRAHAM, LECTURES ON THE SCIENCE
OF HUMAN LIFE, 1872

The desire for good food is as old as time. In the Old Testament, for example, the Israelites look upon wholesome food as a blessing from God as they journey to the Promised Land. But food has not always been revered as such in modern times, particularly in the United States since the Industrial Revolution. The rapid and widespread urbanization that took place in the years following the beginning of industrialization in the U.S. led to a decline in farming, as well as a higher food demand to feed the increasingly populated cities. Even the large agricultural outfits that took over family farms found it difficult to keep up with this demand. The end result was produce and grains stripped of nutrients, canned and packaged goods, and food preservatives for products that had to be transported long distances to "super" markets in urban areas. The stage was thus set for the advent of over-processed foods—a staple of our modern food supply.

Fortunately, today, there are courageous consumers, retailers, manufacturers, and researchers fighting to change the face and direction of nutrition in America. While other industries generally aim to move forward, the prime directive in the health food world, especially in recent years, has been getting "back to the basics." Namely, health food advocates and environmentalists alike have pushed for a return to more natural, sustainable ways of eating and producing food that is untainted by genetically modified organisms (GMOs), pesticides, and other chemicals and additives. This mission has received its share of criticism from Big Agriculture and the bureaucrats, mass-market food industry leaders, and others who make up the anti-health food brigade. Take, for example, the following remarks by a Science Advisor for the U.S. Department of Agriculture (USDA) in 1971:

> Some difficult situations have developed as a result of the recent outburst of enthusiasm for the subject of nutrition and food . . . We regret the opportunity it has given faddists, zealots and other extremists to increase their customers, profits and power structure . . . The indiscriminate distrust of scientific and technological progress that is displayed by such self-appointed guardians of our welfare—guardians who encourage others to be distrustful too—is another hazard in our nutrition and food environment. The surge of interest in buying "natural" and organically grown foods is one manifestation of this distrust . . . The commonly used pesticides about which the extreme environmentalists are so alarmed have undergone much more stringent and extensive testing than the products of food extremists . . . And how do they justify a food production and diet scheme that, if adopted widely, would result in such a reduction of supplies that famine and death would be the fate of so many people?

Incredibly, these ill-informed views continue to be held by many influential people in the food industry, despite the fact that our country and world is burdened with a food supply that is more and more nutritionally empty, frequently contaminated, and controlled by big business and politics. More than ever before, the future of our nutrition, environment, and general health is hinged on a return to sustainable farming techniques, minimal processing, and good old-fashioned natural foods. That is why this chapter offers a look back at the history of our food supply, from early agriculture all the way through industrialization and the rise of modern farming, including the related problems of agricultural politics, food safety, and environmental degradation. At the same time, we'll take a look at some reasons to believe that our food supply has a chance at a more promising future.

A HISTORY OF OUR FOOD SUPPLY: FROM EARLY AGRICULTURE TO THE RISE OF AGRI-BUSINESS

Agriculture, the main source of our food supply, has been essential to human survival since its discovery approximately 10,000 years ago. Humans learned how to domesticate many species of wild food plants as early as 8,000 BC, as farmers cultivated thousands of different strains, each with its own hereditary genetic material, or *germplasm*. The natural vigor and diversity of these plant varieties, which are also known as "land races," allowed for a constant food supply.

In the United States, farming has always been one of the most important industries, and many states rely on agriculture as one of the main sources of income. Over time, however, the industry has undergone dramatic changes, and most of them have occurred in the last 100 years. Today, instead of horse-drawn plows, we have commercial tractors. Rather than pull weeds by hand, it's possible to spray entire fields with herbicides. And while such radical changes have provided many benefits—such as the ability to produce a sufficient food supply for the entire American population—progress has not been uniformly beneficial. Numerous problems exist today, including the destruction of ecosystems and the emergence of food-related illnesses. These problems are all indirect results of changes in agriculture, such as specialization and the growth of farming operations, which occurred following the Industrial Revolution.

The industrialization of agriculture began in the early part of the 1900s and has not stopped since. Before the turn of the twentieth century, the majority of farms were diversified (producing more than a single crop) and farmers took care of their own crops and livestock. Farming was also difficult, laborious work; most of it had to be done manually by farmers and their helpers. But the emergence of concepts such as mechanization, specialization, standardization, and consolidation changed how farms were run for good.

In the early 1900s, farmers started to invest in equipment that would make their job easier. This was also beneficial for the economy, as it meant that money was being spent and products were being sold. Politicians tried to expand upon this trend by promoting specialized agriculture operations, or farms that would act as "experts" on a particular crop (or breed of livestock) and produce only that product. They believed this method would increase efficiency and profitability, and the idea was quickly embraced by farmers.

At the time, the government strongly supported a transformation of agriculture, as the industrial boom had brought about an increased need for manpower in factories. Specialized farming, made easier and more efficient with equipment, freed up a substantial labor force for industry. Few people considered the potential consequences of specialized farming, such as the increased use of chemical fertilizers and pesticides to ensure the highest possible crop yields. According to a project sponsored by Johns Hopkins University, the use of chemicals in agriculture increased more than five times between 1948 and 2008. In addition, the overuse of commercially produced seeds to grow crops has led to erosion and mineral depletion of the soil.

The economy has also felt the impact of specialized farms. Big commercial operations have been able to monopolize their specialty crops and control inflation via pre-determined pricing. Plus, it is inherently risky to depend on only a few farms to produce most of the supply of a certain crop. A single catastrophic event or bad growing season could mean drastic food shortages and skyrocketing prices that might extend to even seemingly unrelated products like cosmetics, pet food, and gasoline.

The consolidation and growth of farms was another and, perhaps, inevitable result of specialization, as farmers' primary goal was to produce the greatest possible amount of crops—a goal that required not only technologically advanced equipment, fertilizers, and pesticides, but also more land. Large-scale operations began to purchase small farms, ultimately leading to the virtual extinction of the latter. According to the 2007 edition of *Structure and Finances of U.S. Farms,* the size of the average farm in the United States has more than doubled since 1950, but less than half as many farms are still in operation. Farms that are larger in size but fewer in number have also exacerbated problems like erosion, pollution, mineral depletion, and reliance on companies that sell genetically engineered seeds.

Despite the problems caused by modern agricultural practices, the farming industry in the U.S. has been seen as efficient and generally successful. Plus, the costs associated with running huge farm operations are low. Nevertheless, there have been numerous "hidden" costs—health risks, environmental damage, and harm to livestock and ecosystems, for example—which is largely due to the fact that agriculture is now dominated by big business. The industry is heavily regulated, with changes and so-called advancements constantly being made and forced upon farmers. Even though public health and the environment should take precedence over profits, the reality is that they often do not. Agricultural policies support maximum profits, production, and shelf life at the expense of our food supply, and as you will see, the effects have been devastating.

AGRICULTURE TODAY

In an interview, Roy Upton RH, DAyu, the Executive Director of the American Herbal Pharmacopoeia, said:

> The manner in which agriculture in this country is practiced is remarkable from an economic and sanitation standpoint and appalling from all health perspectives. Agriculture is clearly a driving economic force . . . with a number of states (such as California) having agriculture among their most profitable industries. Similarly, for the amount of food that is traded in this country it is amazing there are not more outbreaks of illness due to food borne pathogens.

Today, agriculture is a major part of the economy, as it always has been, but it is in dire need of an overhaul. There is always room for improvement, but in order to come up with viable solutions, the impact of a few instrumental factors should be taken into consideration. A few of the most influential forces in the industry today are discussed below.

The Impact of Subsidies and Agricultural Politics

No discussion of agriculture is complete without mentioning agricultural politics and subsidies, which have a huge impact on how U.S.

farms conduct business. Before explaining why subsidizing agriculture is problematic, as well as why agricultural politics are completely illogical, it's important to understand what subsidies are and how they work.

While there are natural health experts who have expounded upon subsidies and their effects (see the inset on page 44), to put it simply, subsidies are funds given to farmers to put towards the operation of their farms. They come in many forms, including cash, cheap crop insurance, price regulations, and incentives. Subsidies might be given to farmers to grow certain crops or raise a specific animal; other times, the farmers may be paid subsidies in return for *not* growing a particular crop. For example, in order to encourage cotton production, farmers may receive subsidies based on their cotton yields. On the other hand, if at some point there is an increased supply of cotton, subsidies may be paid to farmers who choose not to grow cotton at that time.

While subsidies have enabled farmers to survive tough financial times, and given farmers the means to expand and modernize their operations, some government subsidy programs are now outdated. In fact, many programs and policies that were originally implemented under the Lincoln administration still exist today. Among these policies are the Homestead Act, which was enacted in 1862 to encourage the cultivation of more farmland, and the establishment of the USDA. A number of programs have failed to change with the times, as some continue to focus on crops like rice, wheat, soy beans, and corn, which are no longer the most essential commodities. Consequently, billions of dollars have been put into programs that benefit only the largest commercial farms. According to the USDA, "Since 1995, just 10 percent of subsidized farms—the largest and wealthiest operations—have raked in 74 percent of all subsidy payments. Sixty-two percent of the farms in the United States did not collect subsidy payments."

Furthermore, since subsidies are based on yield—because politicians mistakenly believed that such a policy would be effective—farmers set out to obtain the highest yields possible, even if that meant resorting to over-farming (see page 45) or excessive use of industrial-grade chemical fertilizers, pesticides, herbicides, growth hormones, and modified seeds. No one considered that these plants are, in essence, nutritionally useless, that the chemicals contaminate the land and water outside a farm's boundaries, and that people might actually get sick from consuming these products. The only thing that matters is the paycheck.

In other words, subsidies frequently do not go to small farmers who could actually use the money, but huge commercial operations instead, a fact that has been pointed out by the Environmental Working Group (EWG):

> Some 90,000 checks went out to wealthy investors and absentee land owners in more than 350 American cities in 2010, despite the so-called "actively engaged" rule adopted in the 2008 farm bill. This rule is designed to ensure that federal payments go only to those who are truly working the land. It hasn't worked.

In an investigative report published by the *Washington Post*, several wasteful examples were discussed in depth. Here are a few of the highlights:

• "The largest annual subsidy, called direct and countercyclical payments, is given to farmers regardless of what crops they grow—or whether they grow anything at all. The *Post* found that, since 2001, at least $1.3 billion was paid to landowners who had planted nothing since 2000. Among the beneficiaries were homeowners in new developments whose backyards used to be rice fields."

The Conservation Reserve Program

Not all farming subsidies have contributed to the corruption of the agricultural industry, and the Conservation Reserve Program (CRP) is an example. This government program gives farmers money to *idle* farmland—conserve it rather than use it to grow crops—for ten years if it is deemed to be at high-risk for erosion. The Agricultural Adjustment Act (AAA), passed in 1933, was the first piece of legislation to support idling, as farmers were paid subsidies to let fields lie barren in order to drive up farm prices. In 1936, this program was replaced with one that subsidized farmers for planting soil-enriching crops, such as alfalfa, which would not be sold on the market. Unfortunately, programs like these have been eclipsed by unfair subsidies that ultimately harm the environment and small farmers.

- "The multibillion-dollar farm subsidy system often is touted by Congress as a way to save small family farms. Instead, those policies are helping to accelerate their demise, because owners of large farms receive the most subsidies and often use the money to acquire more land."

- "When a maverick Arizona dairyman decided to sell milk for less than the competition, a coalition of giant milk companies and dairies

Subsidies and Our Health

Roy Upton has eloquently summed up how subsidies affect the health of our nation:

On the health side, regulators and legislators are clueless. On one hand, we take tax dollars to subsidize farmers to grow products for the manufacturer of high-fructose corn syrup, one of the greatest contributors to obesity and type 2 diabetes that will eventually lead to greater bankruptcy of the country, pour millions of more tax dollars into campaigns fighting obesity, and then billions into treating diabetes. A large percentage of the food produced in the U.S. is predominately for trade, not eating, is completely wasted, and never even makes it to the compost pile where it can do some good. On the produce side of things, much of our vegetables and fruits are produced in soils that lack essential nutrients necessary for actually creating a nutrient rich food . . . . Soil and crops are force fed with synthetic fertilizers, crops are produced as monocrops. This gives rise to pests requiring the 525 million pounds of pesticides used annually in the U.S. Those pesticides become concentrated in fat cells (linked to obesity), many are carcinogenic, and many contribute to a high rate of reproductive failure. Maybe that is not a bad thing due to overpopulation but really is tragic for the farm workers who have multiple miscarriages and birth defects from pesticide exposure. Perhaps the worst part of our agricultural industrial complex is the many pesticide and pest eradication programs that occur state and federally. Many of these programs (e.g. Light Brown Apple Moth, Medfly) are completely ineffective, costly, expose populations to massive and continued amount of pesticides, and serve no greater purpose than to be used as barriers and incentives for agriculture trade, both state to state and internationally.

decided to crush his initiative. For three years, the milk lobby spent millions on lobbying and campaign contributions and made deals with lawmakers. Congress used a rare procedure to stop the maverick without a hearing."

In sum, agriculture has become a highly commercialized and politics-driven industry in which only a few have power and influence over everyone else. This is worrisome, as a healthy food supply is vital to our survival and well-being. Today, it is being destroyed simply because some people stand to financially benefit. Especially in this tough economic climate, money should not be wasted on subsidizing harmful farming techniques, producing large amounts of marginally worthwhile products, and lining the pockets of those who know how to work the system. But this is exactly what's happening. In 2010 alone, the government spent $96.3 billion on subsidies and programs, most of which benefited the wealthiest large farms. On top of this, few agricultural bills emphasize nutrition, despite the efforts of government agencies to promote healthy eating among parents, children, school administrators, and the general public. When it comes to farming subsidies, health is frequently too expensive to take into account.

Changing a whole system is not easy, though, especially one that is as old and well-established as agriculture. While not all subsidies are bad (see the inset on page 43), allowing business and politics to wield so much power over our most fundamental source of survival in this way will eventually lead to not only massive food shortages, but also land so depleted and stripped of nutrients that farming as we know it will no longer be possible.

Over-Farming

While the widespread availability of advanced farm equipment has allowed for improved productivity and efficiency, mechanization in combination with subsidies has resulted in over-farming, a problem that has snowballed out of control. Excessive farming is part of a vicious cycle: farmers want to maximize their profits by growing as many crops as possible, and government subsidies make their efforts financially worthwhile.

The consequences of this practice have been devastating, particularly for the environment. One famous example is the Dust Bowl of the 1930s, the cause of which can be tracked back to the increased need for food during World War I. To meet the demand, farmers invested in agricultural equipment and heavy machinery that was capable of tilling the land to an extent they had never seen before. Although they succeeded in producing high crop yields, farmers had not foreseen the severe drought that dried out the soil, which had been damaged by over-tilling. When strong windstorms hit, the topmost layer of loosened soil was blown away, resulting in the famous "black blizzards" from which the Dust Bowl takes its name. In some cases, these "blizzards" buried entire homes, farms, barns, and arable land with this dry dirt, turning fertile lands into arid ones.

The election of Franklin D. Roosevelt in 1933 was good news for the environment. In 1935, he established the Soil Conservation Service, which today is a division of the USDA called the Natural Resources Conservation Service (NRCS). The purpose of this agency was to restore the land destroyed by the Dust Bowl, an effort involving the re-introduction of native plants to affected regions, replenishing the top layer of soil with cover crops (see page 58), and planting windbreaks—one or more rows of trees or shrubs designed to block the wind and prevent soil erosion.

The events of the Dust Bowl seem to have been swept under the rug over the past several decades, which may be due to the fact that many subsidies today promote over-farming—the practice that caused the crisis. The main goal of commercial agriculture is quantity, which can be achieved only by purchasing the most advanced equipment, tilling large areas of soil, and growing crops as quickly as possible. And since farms are ever expanding, there is no end in sight for over-farming.

Soil Erosion

In her book *Stolen Harvest* (2000), Vandana Shiva noted that "agricultural cultures, technologies and economies are based on an integration between crops and animal husbandry." In other words, the relationship between crops, animals, and humans is reciprocal—at least it's supposed to be. This natural ecological chain has been disrupted by soil erosion, which has become a problem in many areas of the United States. While most people have heard about soil erosion, the majority probably do not realize that agricultural practices and policies are the underlying cause, or that erosion also affects water, food, whole ecosystems, and even taxes.

The process of erosion involves moving soil through some force, such as water, gravity, or wind. To some extent, this happens naturally. However, modern-day farming methods have dramatically increased the rate at which it occurs so that soil is not being created and replaced quickly enough. Not only is the soil lost, but also everything the soil contains, including earthworms, microorganisms, minerals, fungi, and organic materials that all work together to provide plants with the necessary nutrients and environment. These microorganisms and nutrients strengthen plants and boost their natural resistance to disease and pests. They also provide other living creatures with the essential vitamins and minerals they need to stay healthy.

On February 26, 1937, FDR wrote in his letter from President to Governors, "A nation that destroys its soils destroys itself." This warning should have been heeded at the time, but it was not—and things have not improved since then. In fact, the situation has only become worse. Large areas of soil are so completely over-tilled and depleted of nutrients that nothing is holding it in place anymore. This leaves the soil vulnerable to high rates of erosion, which destroys fertile farmland and increases pollution. In severe cases, *desertification* of once-fertile farmable land can occur. Once desertification takes place, the land is barren and can't be turned back into fertile land. This phenomenon is seen around the world and can almost always be traced back to soil erosion caused by agricultural methods.

If the loss of fertile soil is not sufficient reason to be worried about erosion, the pollution and damage it causes should be. In a 1998 study conducted by the Environmental Protection Agency (EPA) called the National Water Quality Inventory, it was determined that "30 percent of surveyed rivers, 44 percent of surveyed lakes, and 23 percent of surveyed estuaries were contaminated with unsafe levels of nutrient pollution."

Runoff is another problem caused by soil eroison. Also known as sediment, runoff pollutes water and destroys ecosystems due to the fact that once it enters water, it remains stagnant. This reduces the depth of the water and causes it to turn cloudy, effectively killing or reducing populations of fish and other organisms, which has an impact on the environment as a whole. A 2008 study conducted by the EPA and cited by the Grace Communications Foundation stated that "sediment is the most significant non-point source (NPS) pollutant in the U.S." This is a problem for everyone, because NPS pollution does not have a specific origin or source, which is another way of saying that it can come from anywhere and go everywhere. This makes it almost impossible to fight.

Erosion also presents the danger of chemicals entering water systems or the air, since without soil, there is retaining the chemicals that are sprayed on plants or applied directly to fields. Nitrogen and phosphorus from industrial fertilizers are especially dangerous to organisms. According to Robbin Marks, author of *Cesspools of Shame: How Factory Farm Lagoons and Sprayfields Threaten Environmental and Public Health,* "Nitrogen-contaminated groundwater is harmful to humans, particularly to vulnerable populations such as children, the elderly, and people who have suppressed immune systems." This is because nitrogen from fertilizers enters water in the form of nitrates, which is anything but healthy. If small children or babies drink nitrates, a condition known as "blue baby syndrome" may occur, which can cause permanent brain damage and even death. Moreover, the Centers for Disease Control (CDC) have "linked high levels of nitrates in drinking water to spontaneous abortions in women."

Yet another erosion-caused threat to take into consideration is *Pfiesteria piscicida,* which was identified by the EPA in a 2003 report:

> Nutrient pollution is also thought to induce outbreaks of *Pfiesteria.* This toxic dinoflagelate (type of algae) emits a toxin that breaks down the skin tissue of fish, causing bleeding sores or legions. *Pfiesteria* outbreaks have caused major fish kills and are thought to cause memory loss, confusion, respiratory problems, and skin problems in humans.

Even though erosion is not a new phenomenon, agricultural politics and practices continue down the same path, from over-farming lands to over-applying chemicals to fields. Neither money nor politics sufficiently explain this failure or reluctance to change farming techniques. In fact, studies have shown commercial farming practices are actually counter-productive. In an article published by *Science* magazine, David Pimentel revealed that "the loss of soil and water from the U.S. cropland decreases productivity by about $27 billion per year." And yet there have been no real attempts to prevent and stop erosion. However, if it does not stop, we may one day have little or no fertile land left.

Science and research has taught us that soil erosion can be stopped by implementing sustainable farming techniques (see page 56). Why these methods are not enforced or supported in agricultural politics remains a mystery, especially they can effectively slow, delay, or even prevent erosion.

Mineral-Depleted Soils

As you know, the agricultural industry today is largely controlled by big business. Consequently, instead of implementing sustainable farming techniques, farmers work their land with the goal of yielding as many crops as possible. But nature has only so much to give, and soon there will be nothing left to take. This fact has not seemed to register with many commercial farming operations, which use as much fertilizer as is necessary to get crops to grow to their full potential.

The problem with this practice is that plants obtain essential nutrients—which are contained in varying amounts in most fertilizers—through their roots, which means that chemicals entering the soil are absorbed into the plants themselves. The resulting crops appear perfect on the outside, but have little or no nutritional value. In fact, they may actually be harmful when consumed. The rule that we all learned as children—namely, that eating fruits and vegetables is fundamental to good health—is no longer always true today.

The statistics provided in the table on page 50 come from the 1992 Earth Summit regarding mineral depletion of soils around the world. The findings are amazing, but not in a good way.

Since plants require only nutrients, you may be wondering why farmers don't just simply add minerals to the soil rather than fertilizer. The answer is that companies earn huge profits by selling chemical fertilizers, which are inexpensive to produce. In other words, this system is beneficial to farmers and businesses alike, making it even more difficult to enact change.

PERCENTAGE OF MINERAL DEPLETION FROM SOIL DURING THE PAST 100 YEARS, BY CONTINENT			
Continent	**Percentage**	**Continent**	**Percentage**
North America	85%*	Africa	74%
South America	76%	Europe	72%
Asia	76%	Australia	55%

* Some U.S. farms are 100-percent depleted and some are 60-percent depleted; the average is 85-percent depletion as compared to 100 years ago. This is worse than in any other country in the world because of the extended use of fertilizers and "maximum yield" mass-farming methods.

As the saying goes, "You are what you eat." And in today's world, these words are terrifying. Even more terrifying is a statement made by a USDA official in an interview for the 1987 book *Diet for a New America:* "Halting soil erosion and degradation would be prohibitively expensive." To put it another way, the government does not intend to change because to do so would cost too much money.

GMOs and Monoculture

Despite the natural hardiness and versatility of traditional plant varieties, today many growers are abandoning these "land races" in favor of genetically engineered *monocultures,* or single-variety crops grown year after year. This practice has been made possible through the use of GMOs (genetically modified organisms), which have genetically altered seeds with a built-in resistance to environmental factors that can negatively affect crop growth, such as pests. It's said that GMOs produce higher crop yields and provide health benefits, claims that have served to justify their continued use in agriculture. Unfortunately, it isn't the reality.

The true purpose of genetic modification is to improve the appearance and quantity of crops, which comes at the expense of their quality. The problem with GMOs was effectively summarized by Jonathan W. Emord, Esq., an attorney and member of the Certification Board for Nutrition Specialists, who has extensive experience with GM and biotech foods. Emord said:

Fruits and vegetables in American grocery stores today contain lower quantities of nutrients than they did 25 years ago. Modern agricultural practices, quick harvests, preference for larger sized fruits and vegetables, and genetic selection and engineering to favor appearance have contributed to crops that are less nutritious than in prior years. Essential vitamins and minerals have diminished remarkably in some of our most essential staples, including potatoes, tomatoes, bananas, wheat and apples. Take, for example, a potato which is a favorite American vegetable. The average potato has lost nearly 100 percent of its vitamin A, 57 percent of its vitamin C and iron, and 28 percent of its calcium. The same can be said of most "mass produced" foodstuffs. Emphasis today is on storability, appearance and size, and transportability, at the expense of nutritional value.

GMOs and monocultures also have destructive effects on the environment. Clear-cutting across virgin lands destroys natural vegetation, bringing on what is called genetic erosion. By 2050, it's estimated that 25 percent of the world's 250,000 plant species will disappear, and the shift to genetically uniform crops is one of the main contributing factors. In fact, this mass extinction has already started; in Sri Lanka, for example, where farmers grew 2,000 varieties of rice as recently as 1959, there are only five varieties grown there today. And in India, which once boasted 30,000 rice varieties, today more than 75 percent of its total production comes from less than ten varieties. As pointed out in my 1991 *Better Nutrition* article, plant geneticist Jack Harlan warned, "The diversity of our genetic resources stands between us and starvation on a scale we cannot imagine."

In addition to the nutritional and environmental hazards associated with genetically modified monocultures, the practice is also economically unsound. The supply of genetically modified seeds depends on only a few corporations that have monopolized the industry, which could have devastating consequences in the event of an unexpected financial downturn, bad weather, or some other factor resulting in a low or nonexistent seed supply. This problem is compounded by the fact that there are currently no widespread efforts being made to collect non-GMO seeds.

GMOs is a concerning issue, especially since the long-term effects of GM seeds on both humans and animals have not been studied in-depth. In June 2011, an ABC News poll found that 93 percent of Americans are worried about GMOs and want the government to call for mandatory labeling of genetically engineered foods and food ingredients. As of the publication of this book, mandatory labeling has not been implemented.

Pesticides and Pesticide-Resistant Crops

Thanks to the use of GMOs, most crops grown today have a built-in resistance to pests in order to maximize crop yields. Nevertheless, the use of harmful pesticides has only increased. As Bill Freese, an analyst working for the Center for Food Safety, wrote, "The most common type of genetically engineered crops promotes increased use of pesticides, an epidemic of resistant weeds, and more chemical residue in our foods. This may be profitable for the biotech/pesticide companies, but it is bad news for farmers, human health and the environment." According to the Center for Food Safety in 2009, "GE [genetically engineered] crops increased herbicide use by 383 million pounds from 1996 to 2008, with 46 percent of the total increase occurring in 2007 and 2008." These statistics reveal the flaws of the GM approach to agriculture. Since pests have natural adaptive abilities, they are able to build up resistance to pesticides, forcing researchers to re-modify seeds and constantly rework their pesticide formulas and make them more powerful.

The effects of increased pesticide use are far-reaching. Not only do they contaminate the foods we eat, but they also pollute the soil, water, and air. In November 2009, the Center for Food Safety posted the following statement on their website in response to a recent report from the USDA:

Industry claims that GE crops are benefitting the environment ignore the impacts of the over 300+ million additional pounds of pesticides required over the period covered by this study, as well as growing reliance by farmers on high-risk herbicides including 2,4-D and paraquat. In addition to the environmental harm, a report released earlier this year by [The Organic Center] demonstrated that exposure to pesticides is linked to increased risk of reproductive abnormalities, birth defects and neurological problems.

Even non-GMO crops now require more frequent treatments of toxic pesticides due to their increased contact with pesticide-resistant crops. Pesticide use also put pests on the move; driven out of one area, they migrate to another in search for the next food source. This creates a domino effect that forces farmers into a vicious cycle of using stronger and stronger pesticides more and more frequently. Today, there are pests that are immune to virtually every chemical used in pesticides, and they have started to affect yards and hobby gardens.

The overuse of pesticides has made the act of eating even "healthy" foods inherently risky. It has also contaminated groundwater and livestock, as well as caused the death of countless birds, fish, and honeybees.

Terminal Seeds

Little is heard about terminal seeds, or terminator seeds, outside of the agricultural industry, but they are one of the greatest threats to our food supply. Terminal seeds are a type of genetically modified seed that are designed to kill, or "terminate," their own embryos, making them sterile and preventing the growth of the next generation of plants. This ensures that farmers must buy new seeds every year.

Monsanto, an agriculture biotechnology corporation, came under heavy public criticism for the development of their terminator technology, or Varietal Genetic Use Restriction Technologies (V-GURTs), "in which seeds resulting from the first year's planting would be sterile, thereby forcing farmers around the world . . . to buy their seed from them every year rather than saving their best seed for next year's planting," explained SourceWatch.org.

There are fears that Monsanto's "suicide seed" terminator genes might spread to wild plants if they become commercialized (see the inset on page 54). According to Vandana Shiva in *Stolen Harvest*:

After studying these seeds, molecular biologists warned of the possibility of terminator seeds spreading to surrounding crops or to the natural environment—the gradual spread of sterility in seeding plants would result in a global catastrophe that could eventually wipe out higher life forms, including humans.

The Food and Agriculture Organization (FAO) has confirmed this

The Birth and Suspended
Death Sentence of Terminator Seeds

In 1995, D&M International was formed by Monsanto and the Delta Pine and Land Company (D&PL) to market genetically modified cottonseed internationally. The following year, D&PL began to sell insect-resistant cottonseed in the United States. Although an outright merger of Monsanto and D&PL was announced in 1998, it fell through in 1999, which sidetracked D&PL's goal of commercializing the terminator technology developed by Monsanto. Nevertheless, a U.S. patent was issued in early 1998 to both D&PL and the USDA for what was referred to then as a Technology Protection System (TPS), more commonly known as V-GURT or terminator technology.

In a 1998 interview, Willard Phelps, a USDA spokesman, explained that the USDA wanted the technology to be licensed and available to "many seed companies," which some have interpreted to mean agribusiness giants like Monsanto, DuPont, and Dow. Phelps didn't hide the government's reasons for promoting terminator seeds, namely, that they would enable the expansion of genetically modified crops—a central element in their agricultural strategy since the mid-1980s. Moreover, according to GlobalResearch.org, "USDA's Phelps stated that [another] goal in fostering the widest possible development of Terminator technology was 'to increase the value of proprietary seed owned by U.S. seed companies and to open up new markets in Second and Third World countries.'"

In early 1999, D&PL "expressed some desire for further studies of the social and economic implications of their introduction" of terminator seeds. Although Monsanto pledged in 1999 that they would not commercially sell the seeds, the idea has been supported and its industry partners, since the seeds—which must be purchased every year—are great for business.

Other companies, both public and private, have also researched terminator technology. Fortunately, as Vandana Shiva noted in *Stolen Harvest,* as of 2001, "there has been a de facto worldwide moratorium on the use of terminator technology." Just the same, the technology has not been shelved. In fact, an undated USDA publication made no reference to either its ethical or ecological dangers, stating, "In the medium term, the major determinants of the use of [V-] GURT technology will probably be the rapidity with which the technologies can be made robust and the value of the traits that are coupled with these technologies in new crop varieties."

assessment. The FAO Commission on Genetic Resources for Food and Agriculture found that cross-fertilization of crops containing V-GURTs could affect neighboring crops and other plants. Moreover, the fact that "contamination of non-GMO varieties by GMO germplasm has been observed [in North America] . . . suggests that this scenario is a realistic probability."

The Decline of Seed Saving and Heirloom Crops

Heirloom crops are plants with desirable characteristics—such as natural resistance to pests, disease, and extreme weather—that originated before the age of industrialization, when agriculture was still largely subsistence-based. These plants are grown via open pollination, which means their seeds are spread naturally, whether through wind, rain, or insects. Pre-industrial farmers often saved these seeds to use the following year in a practice known as seed saving, which allowed them to continually improve the quality of their crops through careful selection. Seed saving was also highly economical, as it eliminated the need to obtain new seeds year after year.

The introduction of commercially patented, genetically modified seeds, however, has essentially put an end to seed saving. Meanwhile, many heirloom crops are vanishing, and agricultural corporations are becoming more and more powerful. The Center for Food Safety lists 112 lawsuits by Monsanto against individual U.S. farmers for violating patents and contracts by saving seed from one season to the next, which is generally prohibited. According to Monsanto's website:

> Growers who purchase our patented seeds sign . . . an agreement that specifically addresses the obligations of both the grower and Monsanto and governs the use of the harvested crop. The agreement specifically states that the grower will not save or sell the seeds from their harvest for further planting, breeding or cultivation.

Such policies have contributed not only to a monopolized industry, but also a decline in biodiversity among plants, increased nutrient depletion, and more pollution.

Although modern agriculture has failed us in many ways, it can still be restored to a better place. As more people become aware of its problems—rising food prices, food-related illnesses, and environmental ruin—efforts are being made to move towards sustainable farming practices. Furthermore, in an attempt to prevent global disasters, groups are tracking down wild relatives of modern crops in habitats believed to favor their survival. They are also preserving the germplasm of these plant relatives in a global network of gene banks and protected natural sites. Conserving plant diversity, the environment, and our health—indeed, our future—requires us to embrace these safer, sustainable methods.

THE PROMISE OF SUSTAINABLE FARMING PRACTICES

Sustainable agriculture is not a myth. There are already many methods available that can be used to improve the overall quality of the land and crops without having to resort to extensive use of pesticides, strong fertilizers, or genetically engineered seeds. These methods include crop rotation, biodynamic farming, use of heirloom seeds, cover crops, and integrated pest management. Understanding the techniques described in this section is essential for defeating the businesses and lobbyists who advocate the kind of genetically modified farming that is destroying our land, environment, and health.

Crop Rotation

Since farmers want to get the most out of their land, they have a tendency to plant crops whenever possible without allowing the soil to naturally recover from previous plantings. This increases the need for fertilizer, growth hormones, and other chemicals. *Crop rotation*, the practice of alternating between crops grown on a given field, offers an easy solution to this problem.

There are a number of different rotations that farmers can choose. For example, they can grow one crop for a couple years, followed by a year of another crop. Five-year rotation cycles are also possible. Crops that replenish their own nutrient supply and require lower amounts of nutrients to grow—a group that includes soybeans, clover, and legumes—are ideal for in-between plantings.

Crop rotation also naturally decreases the pest population, since pests favor certain crops. By removing that crop for even a single growing season, pests are forced to leave and find a new source of food instead of staying and colonizing the area.

Biodynamic Farming

Biodynamics was developed in the 1920s by Dr. Rudolf Steiner, an Austrian writer, educator, and social activist. The purpose of biodynamic farming is to create an agricultural ecosystem that is balanced, diversified, and mostly self-sustaining. In place of harmful chemicals, preparations consisting of fermented manure, herbs, and minerals are used to vitalize the land, thereby enhancing the quality, nutritional value, and flavor of the crops being cultivated. Biodynamic farmers work in cooperation with other elements in the farm ecosystem, striving to maintain the health of the soil, surrounding plants, and animals.

In essence, biodynamic agriculture is an integrated form of sustainable and organic farming. Using artificially produced chemicals on either the crops or soil is prohibited; only natural growth aids and sources of nutrients such as animal manure and composting are allowed. Biodynamic farming also involves choosing local varieties of crops and livestock, as well as making sure all aspects of the farm benefit each other so that the farm can sustain itself.

Heirloom Seeds

Although saving genetically modified seeds is generally prohibited by patent laws, in the late 1980s, Vandana Shiva started Navdanya, "a movement for saving seed, to protect biodiversity, and to keep seed and agriculture free of monopoly control." According to Shiva, who has since established sixteen seed community seed banks to conserve heirloom seeds, the movement today has "thousands of members who conserve biodiversity, practice chemical-free agriculture, and have taken a pledge to share the seeds and biodiversity they have received as gifts from nature and their ancestors."

In truth, there are seed-saving groups all over the globe, some of which are "official" and others that were informally organized by word of mouth. One such group is the California-based Seed Savers Alliance (see the inset on page 58), which defines itself as "a collective dedicated to saving and sharing seeds among the various gardening communities in Davis. The seed library's mission is to help nurture a

Why Save Seeds?

Seed saving has numerous advantages, which are aptly summed up on the Seed Savers Alliance website:

Humans have been saving seeds for over 12,000 years. However, in our culture much of that knowledge, along with significant biodiversity, has been lost over the last hundred years. When you grow and save your own seeds, you promote seed sovereignty by:

- Increasing the genetic diversity of your own seed stock
- Developing the seed stock that is more resilient and better adapted to our climate and soil
- Perpetuating the knowledge and culture of seed saving
- Providing free seeds to everyone

thriving community of gardeners and seed savers." The alliance also states, "Our vision is to establish a seed library and seed garden to provide free access to seeds and seed saving knowledge to everyone. We support gardeners and seed savers, from beginner to expert, through the process of growing, harvesting, and saving seeds."

When stored properly, heirloom seeds can be saved for years without taking up much space. It is crucial to save these seeds, which are ever evolving and naturally adapt to the environment. This ensures a food supply that is easier and less costly to produce, as well as more varied, nutritious, and flavorful.

Cover Crops

Cover crops are plants that may be grown for conservation-related purposes such as reducing erosion, increasing biodiversity and organic matter, absorbing and redistributing nutrients in the soil, suppressing weeds, or protecting growing crops from damage. As you may recall, cover crops were planted as one way of remedying the severe environmental problems caused by the Dust Bowl.

Cover crops may not be new, but they have fallen by the wayside in recent decades as commercial farming took over. Today, many farmers are trying to re-implement cover crops but lack sufficient know-how, which has been pointed out by the Department of Horticulture and Crop Science at Ohio State University:

> Recent environmental and ecological awareness has started a resurgence in cover crop use. Although cover crops have been used for centuries, today's modern farmer has grown up in a generation which has replaced the use of cover crops with widespread use of fertilizers and herbicides. Now as some farmers are trying to use cover crops, they lack the information and experience to be successful. University and private researchers are going back to the basics and are experimenting with beneficial plants to determine how they can best be used in modern farming practices to supplement or replace purchased inputs.

Yet, the practice of growing cover crops is relatively simple, and there is a wide range of traditional cover crops from which farmers can choose, including oats, buckwheat, winter rye, winter wheat, white clover, and sweet clover. There are crop options for practically any time of the year, which means cover crops will not interfere with the prosperity of farms; they can simply be planted after a harvest to replenish unused fields. Planting cover crops is also a natural way to reduce the need for herbicides and fertilizers, because rich soil almost always contains beneficial insects and microbes, which prevent crop-pest infestations. If the soil quality is high, there is little need for industrial-grade fertilizers.

Integrated Pest Management

Also referred to as "IPM," integrated pest management harnesses the natural interactions between pests, natural enemies, and the surrounding environment in order to control pests. This may involve introducing a non-destructive natural predator, or growing pest-resistant plants along with the main crop in order to keep pests from threatening the harvest. Preventing crop pests from infesting fields is also an important aspect of IPM. Taking the appropriate action by, for example, minimizing weeds before the problem gets out of hand eliminates the need for harmful chemical pesticides.

Some states, such as Minnesota, have been more proactive than others when it comes to improving agricultural practices that promote sustainability. In 1987, Minnesota established the Energy and Sustainable Agriculture Program (ESAP) to support sustainable agricultural techniques and programs, as well as to ensure that all Minnesota agriculture is "based on dynamic, flexible farming systems that are profitable, efficient, productive, and founded on ethics of land stewardship and responsibility." According to the state's Department of Agriculture, the program also aims to "strive to understand and respect the complex interconnectedness of living systems, from soil to people, so as to protect and enhance all natural resources for future generations." This is achieved through workshops, free educational materials, a low-interest shared savings loan program, and assistance to farmers who adopt organic farming.

Minnesota also implemented the Minnesota Grown Program, a partnership between the state's Department of Agriculture and producers of specialty crops and livestock, to support farms that sell locally. It was started by specialty crop growers to differentiate their produce from that of competitors located thousands of miles away. The program now has 1,100 members, which include farmers' markets, CSA farms (Community Supported Agriculture), wineries, meat processors, livestock producers, garden centers, pick-your-own farms, Christmas tree growers, fruit and vegetable planters, and producers of honey, wild rice, maple syrup, cheese, and gourmet products.

States like California, Hawaii, and New York have also been proactive. Some of the most promising projects include the Agricultural Enterprise Park, which is currently being planned by farmers, nonprofit groups, and local politicians in Suffolk County, New York. There is also a hydroponic greenhouse under construction for Hudson Valley Produce Farms. These projects, along with many others (see the inset on page 63), have a common goal of bringing new life to local agriculture by advocating locally grown foods and supporting small farms that focus on sustainability.

The effectiveness of these programs should inspire other states to follow their lead. If similar projects were undertaken on a large-scale, not only would farms (and the soil) benefit, but also anyone who eats the food grown on these farms. Focusing on local farms and locally grown produce also reduces the need to transport and preserve foods for lengthy periods of time. This, in turn, decreases the use of fossil fuels—which are used by trucks to transport crops—and eliminates the need for chemical preservatives and genetically engineered crops with a long shelf life.

As recently as March 2012, the American Farmland Trust called upon Congress to take more progressive measures to improve agriculture, energy, food, and the environment. Among other goals, the Trust called for a reduction in the government's role in farmland loss, protection and support for food system programs, and a bigger role for agriculture in decreasing greenhouse gases. The group also wants to involve farmers in efforts to improve water quality, create "Farmers Corps" that encourages new farmers, and give schools and low-income consumers better access to locally grown foods.

There have also been efforts at the global level. The Center for Sustainable Development (CENESTA), for example, is a non-governmental organization (NGO) dedicated to sustainable community- and culture-based development that represents small-scale farmers and consumers. CENESTA's Maryam Rahmanian has spoken of the importance of "agro-ecology," which the group defines as "small-scale business which stems from local farmers' know-how and scientific research in order to develop processes which stem from a social and cultural perspective." Rahmanian also described this concept as "not a market-niche, not a way to feed large groups of business people, but a way to feed the small-scale consumer." In an interview for Soroptimist International, an organization that works on behalf of women worldwide, she said that CENESTA fights for those who are excluded from land ownership by big businesses that use it for farming and mining. Very often, the land they are allocated is commercially not viable.

Agro-ecology is a key tool for bolstering the resilience of small farmers. Now it's a question of how to turn a community-based concept into a global movement. Many believe that this is a mission in which the FAO's Committee on World Food Security (CFS) should take a more active role. Groups have also asked the UN Framework Convention on Climate Change (UNFCCC) to pay more attention to food security, trade rules, and genetic resources, which are all important aspects of agro-ecology. As Olivier de Schutter, UN Special Rapporteur on the Right to Food, explained to Soroptimist International at the Committee on World Food Security in October 2012, "[Agro-ecology] is also important so that farmers can adapt to climate change—it will improve the health of the soil and enhance agro-diversity."

According to Soroptimist International, the following obstacles must be removed in order for these global efforts at sustainability to be successful:

- Bias of policymakers against small farms in favor of big business.

- Agricultural policies that are shaped by requirements of export markets.

- Lack of secure access to land for small farmers, which makes them less willing to invest in the land by, for example, implementing erosion projects.

- Focus on biotechnology leading to major investments in corn and wheat production over agro-ecology, which is less lucrative.

The success of agro-ecology and collectives depends on international cooperation and commitment. As of the publication of this book, various groups have been encouraged to find multi-stakeholders who are willing to work for these issues, thereby forcing policymakers to take agro-ecology more seriously.

Consumers play a key role in restoring agriculture and our diets to a better place. If more individuals were aware of how big business affects our environment and food supply and demanded change, farmers might be more inclined to adopt sustainable, organic practices. Consumers have more power than they realize when it comes to making their voices heard. Since they are the ones who ultimately control how their money is spent, they can choose to support local farms that use more environmentally and nutritionally friendly agricultural techniques, in turn persuading more farms to at least consider such methods.

Farmers, too, must learn to look past the dollar and recognize how modern farming practices are negatively impacting the environment, our food, and consequently, our health. Of course, no one wants to begrudge farmers their livelihood; but for the good of the economy, the planet, and the well-being of the entire population, there should be more focus on sustainable agriculture and less reliance on detrimental government subsidies.

"Slow" Food

Despite the dismal state of agriculture and the food industry as a whole, in the last few decades, there have been some positive developments in our relationship with and respect for food. One such development is the "slow food" movement, which is the polar opposite of fast-food culture. According to Slow Food USA, the U.S. branch of the organization started in 1989, slow food is "an idea, a way of living and a way of eating. It is part of a global, grassroots movement with thousands of members in over 150 countries, which links the pleasure of food with a commitment to community and the environment." Slow Food USA's mantra is:

Good: The word good can mean a lot of things to a lot of people. For Slow Food, the idea of good means enjoying delicious food created with care from healthy plants and animals. The pleasures of good food can also help to build community and celebrate culture and religious diversity.

Clean: When we talk about clean food, we are talking about nutritious food that is as good for the planet as it is for our bodies. It is grown and harvested with methods that have a positive impact on our local ecosystems and promotes biodiversity.

Fair: We believe that food is a universal right. Food that is fair should be accessible to all, regardless of income, and produced by people who are treated with dignity and justly compensated for their labor.

Another important organization is Oldways Preservation and Trust, which was founded in 1990 by the late K. Dun Gifford. Oldways describes itself as a program to "help consumers improve their food and drink choices, encourage traditional sustainable food choices, and promote enjoyment of pleasures of the table."

CONCLUSION:
THE FUTURE OF OUR FOOD SUPPLY

An estimated 8.3 billion people will walk the globe by the year 2030. To feed a population this large, the FAO predicts that farmers will have to grow nearly 30 percent more grain than they do today, increasing demands on the soil. "Taking the long view," geologist David Montgomery told *National Geographic*, "We are running out of dirt."

It's clear that agriculture has a long way to go before it will be in a good place. But as we have seen, more efforts are being made in communities around the world to emphasize the importance of growing healthy, sustainable foods. Although there will always be people who seem unconcerned about drug-enhanced livestock and GMOs, and who refuse to see that a business-as-usual approach to agriculture is endangering our food supply, one fact is simply indisputable; namely, modified foods, monocultures, and over-farming have done more harm than good. As Roy Upton stated:

It took a New York district court to demand that the FDA stop the indiscriminate use of 28.8 million pounds of antibiotics that are used in raising animals that will grace the kitchen table of most Americans—a practice that is estimated to lead to resistant strains of bacteria that kill 99,000 Americans every year.

And as John Robbins wrote in his 2001 book, *The Food Revolution:*

When you choose to affirm the dignity inherent in life and to uphold the beauty, the magic, and the mystery of the living Earth, something happens. It happens whether or nor anyone else recognizes your efforts, and it happens regardless of how wounded and flawed you are. What happens is you join the long lineage of human beings who have stood for and helped to bring about a future worthy of all the tears and prayers our species has known. Your life becomes a statement of human possibility. Your life becomes an instrument through which a healthier, more compassionate, and more sustainable future will come to be.

3

Politics, the FDA, and Your Health Choices

The Great Health Freedom Battles in U.S. History

"No surrender! No retreat!"

—MAX HUBERMAN

As you read in the first two chapters, there were few standards in place for food purity, water safety, and public health in the late nineteenth and early twentieth centuries. The decades leading up to the creation of the Food and Drug Administration (FDA), which was established by the Food and Drug Act of 1906, were largely characterized by disease, food contamination, and filth in the United States, especially in cities. At the same time, the U.S. food supply was increasingly bereft of nutrients that were much needed by the Depression-era population, a situation made worse by the overuse of poisonous insecticides. Lax or nonexistent standards for public health, in combination with rising agribusiness, resulted in a nation whose health was at risk.

A man who was keenly aware of this problem was Harvey Wiley, a doctor who later emerged as a health crusader and vocal supporter of food and drug regulations. As the first leader of the FDA, Wiley proved to be not only the country's strongest and most visionary consumer safety advocate, but also the agency's most enduring critic. As you will see, the FDA quickly drifted away from the precedents set by Wiley, and moved toward institutional opposition to supplements and natural health products. This chapter traces this unfortunate evolution, and reveals how an agency that was originally intended to protect public health is now one of its greatest obstacles.

HOW WE GOT HERE: BACKGROUND ON THE FDA

To give even the briefest overview of the FDA, we have to take a look at Dr. Harvey Wiley, the agency's courageous first leader. According to a 2006 edition of *FDA Consumer:*

> In the 1880s, when Wiley began his 50-year crusade for pure foods, America's marketplace was flooded with poor, often harmful products. With almost no government controls, unscrupulous manufacturers tampered with products, substituting cheap ingredients for those represented on labels: Honey was diluted with glucose syrup; olive oil was made with cottonseed; and "soothing syrups" given to babies were laced with morphine. The country was ready for reform . . . and for Wiley.

Born in a log farmhouse in Indiana in 1844, Wiley was a top graduate of Hanover College in 1867, and in 1871, received a medical degree from the then new Medical College of Indiana. After earning a degree in chemistry from Harvard University in 1873, he underwent a period of intense study there, after which he accepted a faculty position in Purdue University's chemistry department in 1874. Four years later, he moved to Germany to continue his research on food science and nutrition at the Imperial Food Laboratory in Bismark. Upon his return to Indiana in 1879, and with the help of the Indiana State Board of Health, Wiley began "a study of the adulteration of sugar by the addition of glucose and published a report to the [board] in 1881," wrote William and Carter in their two-volume *The E-Z Encyclopedia of Food Controversies and the Law.*

In 1882, the Commissioner of Agriculture, George Loring, offered Wiley the position of Chief Chemist at the USDA, since he wanted someone who could objectively approach the study of potential food ingredients and additives. Due in large part to Wiley's work as Chief Chemist, several pure-foods bills were introduced in Congress throughout the 1880s and 1890s. Unfortunately, all of them were ultimately tossed out thanks to powerful lobbyists, as well as a few key industry apologists in the government.

After addressing questions posed by Congress regarding the safety of chemical preservatives used in foods, Wiley was awarded a grant of $50,000—the equivalent of approximately $1.25 million today—in

1902 to "study the effects of a diet consisting, in part, of the various preservatives." To bring his cause to the public, Wiley organized a group of healthy young male volunteers, later known as the "Poison Squad," to serve as human subjects in experiments testing the effects of chemicals and adulterated foods. The end result was the Pure Food and Drugs Act, which was signed into law by President Theodore Roosevelt on June 30, 1906. The bill was largely written by Wiley, who was then appointed to oversee its administration. As the first leader of the Food and Drug Administration, he was a coalition builder and crusader for national food and drug regulation, which earned him the sobriquet, "Father of the Pure Food and Drugs Act." Still, as it was written in *FDA Consumer,* "The battle had been won—but not the war."

Over the course of his career, Wiley tangled with enemies inside and outside of government. He even clashed with President Roosevelt, who was angered by Wiley's condemnation of saccharin, which the president liked to take with his tea. Wiley also openly called for the reversal of twenty-four food and drug approval decisions relating to food nutrition issues, such as artificial preservatives and colors, benzoate of soda, labeling of corn syrup, the composition of evaporated milk and, of course, saccharin.

In 1912, Wiley resigned from this position and took over the laboratories of the Good Housekeeping Research Institute, the product-evaluation contingent of the magazine. Here he worked ceaselessly on behalf of American consumers, establishing the "Good Housekeeping Seal of Approval." According to *FDA Consumer,* in his nineteen years heading up the Institute's laboratories, Wiley "led the fight for tougher government inspection of meat; for pure butter unadulterated with water; and for whole wheat flour, which growers were mixing with other grains."

One year before his death, Wiley penned a work entitled, *The History of a Crime Against the Food Law: The Amazing Story of the National Food and Drugs Law Intended to Protect the Health of the People, Perverted to Protect Adulteration of Foods and Drugs.* The book was a blistering indictment of what he saw as the corporation-influenced bastardization and emasculation of the Food and Drugs Act. According to Royal Lee (see page 68), "Truly, as Dr. Wiley sadly remarked in his book . . . the makers of unfit foods have taken possession of Food and Drug enforcement, and have reversed the effect of the law, protecting the criminals that adulterate foods, instead of protecting the public health."

Wiley's final years were spent fighting the battle against the adulteration of refined sugar. He died in 1930 at the age of eighty-six and was buried at Arlington National Cemetery in Washington, DC, leaving behind a legacy defined by truth, consumer safety, and good science—a legacy that the FDA has thus far not upheld.

THE FDA'S SHAMEFUL RECORD: FROM 1930 TO 1980

The year 1930 not only marks the death of one of the greatest health advocates of the modern era; it also marks the rough beginning of the FDA's campaign against health freedom. The span of time covered in this section was the first wave of the agency's assault on nutritional supplements and other health freedom issues.

The Persecution of Royal Lee

One person who took Harvey Wiley's legacy to heart was Royal Lee, DDS, who was born on April 7, 1895 and raised on a farm in southwestern Wisconsin. According to Mark Anderson, who runs the website DrRoyalLee.com, "Lee forever approached humanity's problems in a practical way." In his lifetime, Lee, the president of Lee Engineering, had over seventy mechanical and electrical devices patented. In fact, "the badges of his company . . . could be found in almost any device of advanced technology, and there was probably no field in industry—from automotive to military to agriculture to the U.S. space program—that did not rely on one of his inventions."

Yet, despite his success in the engineering field, from early childhood, Lee's greatest love and interest had always been nutrition. By age twelve, he had compiled a comprehensive "notebook on biochemistry and nutrition by copying definitions from the school dictionary," wrote David Morris, an osteopathic doctor. By the time he was sixteen, Lee was buying books on physiology and biochemistry, and keeping a notebook filled with "pertinent data." He was particularly fascinated with the endocrine system, which he believed was the "master control mechanism" of the body. In 1916, at the age of twenty-one, Lee began developing a concentrate that would optimize endocrine health by delivering all known vitamins and minerals in their natural bioactive state.

After serving overseas in the U.S. Army during World War I, Lee graduated from Marquette University Dental College in Milwaukee and shocked his professors with a bombshell graduation paper entitled, "The Systemic Cause of Dental Caries." Based on documented research, the paper argued that the true cause of tooth decay is bodily dysfunction resulting from malnutrition and resulting endocrine system problems. Lee did not pursue dentistry after graduation, however, as he was more interested in developing dental instruments, which led him to engineering.

Meanwhile, in the 1920s, America was facing a new threat: coronary heart disease. Lee believed that the condition was related to nutritional deficiency, since foods like flour and rice were stripped of vitamins and other nutrients via commercial processing. Putting his engineering know-how to work, Lee designed and fabricated devices to extract nutrients and concentrate food without heating or mechanically refining it. By 1929, he had invented the "world's first raw, whole-food supplement," which he called Catalyn, "over half a century before 'raw' and 'whole-food' [had] even entered the public discussion about nutrition," wrote Mark Anderson. Lee's Vitamins Product Company, which today is called Standard Process, was born.

Lee began to sell Catalyn after it was given positive reviews by many doctors. According to Karl B. Lutz, the supplement "was sold with a statement that it 'produces results in two ways—by regulation of metabolism (an immediate effect), and by building up the vitality and resistance.'" The circular included with the product read, "We earnestly request that if you have any of the diseases or conditions listed below, you consult your physician as to the advisability of using Catalyn either alone or as a supplementary treatment according to the schedules given."

In 1934, the FDA brought a federal suit against Dr. Lee and his new company, which went to trial in 1939. According to the FDA, Catalyn was "misbranded" because the "consensus of medical opinion" was that it was not effective against the conditions for which it was recommended. At the trial, however, there were numerous testimonials as to the product's health benefits. In fact, as Lutz reported, there was "not a shred of evidence that Catalyn had ever had any bad effects on anyone." Nevertheless, the agency had the full support of the government, and Lee lost the case. Later, when a second lawsuit was brought against him in 1962, he pleaded no contest and accepted a consent decree. According to Lutz, "It can be easily understood that Dr. Lee foresaw a second trial weighted against him on the ground of an antiquated 'consensus of medical opinion.'"

It's been widely speculated that the real reason for the FDA's venomous persecution of Dr. Lee is that he had been—and continued to be—a "most vocal critic of the manner in which the FDA had departed from the principles of Dr. Harvey Wiley." After all, it was Lee who re-published Wiley's *The History of a Crime Against Food Law,* believing that the public deserved to know the true history of the FDA. Karl Lutz wrote that this act was "the equivalent of high treason in the minds of the FDA bureaucrats."

Clinton Ray Miller, who headed the National Health Federation (NHF) and was one of the leaders in the fight for the Hosmer-Proximire Vitamin Bill (see page 71), said in his testimony to Congress, "Dr. Lee's cardinal 'sin' against the FDA was to publish the truth about the criminal takeover of that agency, and widely disseminate information which carefully documented the deplorable national malnutrition rampant in the U.S."

The FDA Raids

As early as the 1950s, the FDA began to take advantage of a 1948 court order (*Kordel v. United States*) for the purpose of expanding the definition of product labeling to include any materials, such as flyers, given out or sold by a health food maker to promote its products. The FDA started to exert increasing pressure on health food stores and manufacturers by claiming that certain health products were "misbranded," a tactic that led to the seizure of certain health products by the FDA or other federal agents.

Beginning in the 1960s, the FDA tried to expand the definition of labeling to include books as well. In December 1960, government agents entered the warehouses of the Balanced Foods Company in New York City and seized copies of *Folk Medicine* and *Arthritis and Folk Medicine,* two popular works by the late doctor D. C. Jarvis. They also confiscated bottles of vinegar and honey, which Jarvis frequently referenced in his books. The FDA brought a suit against Balanced Foods in New York's Federal District Court on the grounds that its vinegar and honey products constituted "misbranded drugs." Famed industry attorney, Milton Bass, won the case for Balanced Foods and the health food industry, but this was only the beginning.

Throughout the 1960s, the FDA used inspectors to illegally "bug" health food retailers and manufacturers. During a 1961 FDA inspection of American Health (then called American Dietaids), a hidden tape recorder carried by an inspector malfunctioned, revealing its presence to company officials. Nevertheless, the practice continued and would later be acknowledged in sworn testimony at a Senate subcommittee hearing on administrative practices and procedures in 1965. Even then, raids continued into the early 1990s (see the insets 72, 78, and 80).

The Vitamin Volstead Act and the Hosmer-Proxmire Vitamin Bill

In Chapter One, it was mentioned that the American Medical Association (AMA) tried to run its competition out of town with the Flexner Report of 1910, which aimed to limit school accreditation only to medical institutions that taught allopathic (drug- and surgery-based) medicine. According to Eleanor McBean, in 1911, Dr. W. A. Evans, one of the leading mainstream medical "bosses" and Chicago health commissioner gave these instructions to physicians at the annual AMA convention:

> The thing for the medical profession to do, is to get right into, and man every important health movement; man health departments, tuberculosis societies, housing societies, child care and infant societies, etc. The future of the profession depends on it . . . The profession cannot afford to have these places occupied by other medical men.

By the 1960s, the AMA had allegedly created a division called the Department of Investigations to identify and suppress any type of alternative approach that challenged mainstream medicine. The department, which consisted of at least seventy people, worked to deny practitioners of chiropractic medicine, podiatry, and many other alternative therapies access to the healthcare system.

PART 1 ■ FDA Raids and Abusive Tactics

In April 2007, NaturalNews.com ran an article by writer Mike Adams entitled, "Tyranny in the USA: The True History of FDA Raids on Healers, Vitamin Shops, and Supplement Companies." He discusses the raids of Life Extension, an organization dedicated to anti-aging, that took place in February 1987. This raid serves as one such example of the FDA-orchestrated "campaigns of terror."

According to Adams, on February 26, 1987, more than twenty armed FDA agents and U.S. Marshals stormed the offices of the Life Extension Foundation (LEF), located in Fort Lauderdale, Florida. Simultaneously, another group of FDA agents entered the LEF warehouse, detaining William Faloon, the Foundation's founder, at gunpoint. They searched the employees, who were lined up against the wall, and confiscated thousands of items, including dietary supplements, office files, and over 5,000 copies of the LEF newsletter.

Instead of submitting to the FDA as they had been advised, Faloon and the Life Extension Foundation chose to fight for their First Amendment rights. As LEF officer Saul Kent explained, the group "decided to wage all-out war against the FDA. We did this knowing that we would not only risk our livelihood, but our personal freedom as well."

The FDA, in conjunction with other federal agencies, ultimately filed fifty-six criminal charges against Kent and Faloon. After an eleven-year reign of terror and millions of taxpayer dollars, the attempted prosecution failed, and LEF prevailed. As Adams stated in his article, it was the first time in eighty-eight years that the FDA had been forced to throw in the towel. Saul Kent commented that, "The FDA's dismissal of the charges against me [and Bill Faloon] is an unprecedented victory against FDA tyranny that goes far beyond winning in court. The FDA's historic defeat is a victory for everyone who cherishes freedom in healthcare."

In 1994, the Life Extension Foundation established the "FDA Holocaust Museum" to expose how, according to the Foundation, "an incompetent and corrupt bureaucracy has caused millions of humans to needlessly suffer and die."

Just prior to their establishment of this division, in January 1959, the AMA approached the FDA to request the agency drastically limit the potencies of most vitamins by reclassifying and regulating them as prescription drugs. Clinton Ray Miller later said that the "FDA dutifully issued their 'AMAish' vitamin regulations in June 1962," waiting until 1968 to schedule hearings on these initially proposed regulations, which intended to bar all but eight vitamins and four minerals, and strictly enforce dosages. Loud protests from consumers forced the FDA to amend these regulations; but even the adjusted guidelines allowed access only eleven vitamins and six minerals, which, according to the NHF's Kirkpatrick W. Dilling, would be "strictly limited as to quantity, [and] 40 or more other nutrients [would be] arbitrarily . . . banned."

As explained by Frank Murray in *More Than One Slingshot*, "Since the FDA was convinced that the American diet provided ample vitamins and minerals, the agency undertook to prevent manufacturers of vitamin and mineral supplements [from implying] that their products might help to maintain good health." Murray added:

Thus, acting as Big Brother, the FDA felt justified in taking steps to prevent consumers from purchasing "useless" dietary supplements, especially in health food stores. In that regard the FDA would have required that labels on vitamin and mineral supplements carry this warning: "Vitamins and minerals are supplied in

---

The Quackbusters Quack the Loudest

The 1960s were contentious years in the health freedom arena. On October 25, 1965, the FDA and AMA held a so-called "National Conference on Medical Quackery" in the nation's capital to combat what it called the promoting of "worthless pills." Less than two miles away, however, the National Conference on Health Monopoly was convened by the California-based National Health Federation (NHF), which denounced the "unholy alliance" between the AMA and the FDA.

The opening speaker at the NHF conference, Dr. Miles Robinson, told *The Evening Star,* "The AMA and its friends want to sell the public on the preposterous idea that everything wrong with it can be fixed up with a pill. A pill for constipation; a pill for headache; a pill for tennis elbow; a pill to calm you down; a pill to pop you up." He continued, "Talk about medical quackery! Talk about the gullible public being taken in! Never in the history of the world has there been such quackery on such a wholesale, and respectable appearing, scale!"

---

abundant amounts by commonly available foods. Except for persons with special medical needs, there is no scientific basis for recommended routine use of dietary supplements." Testimony and evidence presented at the hearings clearly disproved the FDA claims on which the [proposed] regulations were based.

Led by Utah Congressman David King and the National Dietary Foods Association—which would later become the National Nutritional Foods Association (NNFA)—American consumers were able to beat back these regulations at first, but they kept resurfacing in various forms over the next decade.

On December 14, 1972, the FDA published a "Proposed Statement of Policy" related to vitamins A and D, which would have instantly banned multivitamin supplements with more than 10,000 international units (IU) of vitamin A and 400 IU of vitamin D. At the time, vitamin A supplements typically varied between 10,000 and 50,000 IU, and vitamin D supplements usually provided anywhere from 1,000 to 10,000 IU; in other words, vitamin D would have been eliminated from the market, and sale of vitamin A would have been limited to very low-dose supplements.

Still, this was not all the FDA intended with the proposal. The actual underlying goal was to use the "druggification" of two very basic vitamins as a regulatory Trojan horse, in turn allowing the agency to impose similarly arbitrary and capricious regulations on most, if not all, other supplements. Ignoring legal challenges to the FDA, Commissioner Alexander Schmidt issued "final" vitamin regulations immediately upon taking office in 1972. The so-called Final Regulations of August 1973 "embodied all of the regulatory theories of the previous FDA administration," which were, of course, faulty.

Taken as a whole, the regulations issued by the FDA after the hearings were designed to classify vitamins and minerals with more than 150 percent of the already incredibly low Recommended Daily Allowance (RDA) levels as prescription drugs. Many referred to the regulations as the "Vitamin Volstead Act" to highlight the parallels between the regulations and the Volstead Act, the legislation responsible for Prohibition in the early twentieth century.

To stem the tide of the FDA's increasingly out-of-control and irrational proposals, and to tackle the all-out "Vitamin Prohibition" push led by the FDA and its medical establishment apologists, in 1973 Wisconsin Senator William Proxmire introduced S-2801, or the Food Supplement Amendment of 1973. Also called the Proxmire Amendment and the Hosmer-Proxmire Vitamin Bill, it was the Senate counterpart to the HR-643/HR-6043 bill introduced in the House of Representatives by California Congressman Craig Hosmer. This landmark legislation, which was introduced in several different versions in both houses of Congress, was meant to prevent the FDA from classifying vitamins and minerals as drugs, and to require the agency to regulate them as foods or food supplements.

Testimony from leaders in Congress and the health industry (see the inset below) given in the "Vitamin, Mineral and Diet Supplement" hearings in October 1973 was truly damning to the FDA's case. At the time, FDA Commissioner Schmidt said, "Few programs have created greater public discussion. The controversy continues to this moment. Tens of thousands of letters have been written to the FDA and to Con-

---

Voices of the FDA Hearings

In addition to Congressman Hosmer and Senator Proxmire, there were a few stand-out stars of the FDA proceedings, including Milton Bass, Clinton Ray Miller, and Max Huberman, who were at the vanguard of what we might call the "Truth Brigade." The power and truth of their remarks helped sway Congress to act in favor of the American people.

Congressman Craig Hosmer (1915–1982). A decorated U.S. Navy Rear Admiral who served as a congressman in California from 1953 to 1974, Hosmer is responsible for introducing the House's counterpart to the Proxmire legislation. In his testimony before the FDA, he stated:

> [Where] particular vitamins or minerals have never been shown to be harmful when taken in quantities even grossly in excess of [RDAs], then there is absolutely no justification for defining them as drugs, which then can be made subject to prescription. In answer to this, the FDA will tell you that it has no intention of requiring prescriptions for non-harmful food supplements. But I ask you: Have you ever heard of giving a bureaucrat power

---

he did not eventually use? Of course not . . . The FDA should not ask for power it does not need for the protection of the public, and all that the bills before us propose to do is to put out of FDA's reach for power that which it was grasping, but does not need.

Congressman Philip Crane (1930–). Crane served as a distinguished Illinois legislator from 1969 to 2004, including the period of time during which the state produced some of the greatest supplement advocates rather than critics. At the FDA hearings, he remarked, "The legislation before us places the burden of proof upon those who seek to limit our freedom, and it takes from those who seek to use that freedom in a manner they believe is consistent with the public interest."

Milton Bass (1921–2000). According to Bob Ullman, an attorney for a prestigious New York law firm and one of his colleagues for nearly forty years, Bass "had a passion for the law and vast intellectual capabilities." Ullman also said, "He loved the challenge and was able to take on a cause through the highest courts." Bass, who fought for the passage of the Hosmer-Proximire Vitamin Bill for over a decade, offered powerful testimony at the hearings:

> We are faced with an attempt by the [FDA] to tell the American people what they can eat and how much they can eat, totally aside from any question of safety . . . We do not believe that the FDA should be able to bar or restrict the sale of the product just because it believes you do not need to or that you would be better off eating oatmeal. This Bill is essential for the protection of the public . . . This Bill involves the protection of individual freedom. The public interest is clear. There is no valid reason for the interference with the individual's freedom by the FDA to impose its beliefs and desires . . . We earnestly request this Committee to support H.R. 643 as a necessary protection for individual freedom and a stop sign on over-regulation.

Clinton Ray Miller (1922–). A political activist, Miller began his career in Utah in the 1950s, where he defeated proposals for water fluoridation eight times. He then went to Washington, DC, in 1962, where he played a pivotal role in the passage of the Kefauver Harris Amendment, which requires informed consent from human subjects of experimental treatments, as well as full disclosure of potential risks and side effects. As executive director of the National Health

Federation (NHF), he led the organization's "Congress on Health Monopoly" conferences in the 1960s, bringing national attention to the "unholy alliance" between the FDA and the pharmaceutical and medical establishment, most notably the AMA. The conferences also exposed the inherent hypocrisy of the "National Conference on Medical Quackery" co-sponsored by the FDA and AMA that was held around the same time (see the inset on page 73).

In October 1973, Miller gave his remarks at the hearings to "curb the U.S. [FDA's] regulatory attempt to over-extend its power over our diets where safety or fraud are not at issue." He also said:

> We are as sensitive about intrusions on our health freedoms as others are when their religious freedoms are threatened or trampled. We demand the right to choose our own doctor or diet. So, naturally, we were outraged when FDA proposed to dictate our diet . . . We have given voice to those soil, nutritional, and environmental scientists who advocate exercise, pure air, pure water and the gentle nutritional pathway to health by concentrating, selecting, and combining nutrients and drugless therapies which, admittedly, represent an economic threat to the harsher and more expensive therapies and theories they challenge.

Max Huberman (1921–2008). The health food store that Max started with his wife, Ruth, in 1958 was one of the first in the nation to sell organic produce and stayed in business for thirty-three years. According to Huberman's son, Mark, "In 1972, my father was elected to his first of an unprecedented five terms as president of the [NNFA] at a pivotal time in the growth of the health food industry. Under his leadership, NNFA made organic foods and environmentalism industry priorities." Huberman's motto was always, "No surrender! No retreat!" and he was an instrumental figure in the battle for the Hosmer-Proximire Bill. As president of the NNFA, he testified at the hearings, saying:

> For the past forty years health food retailers have been providing the only nutritional alternative to the thousands of empty-calorie, overly processed convenience foods that crowd the shelves of markets across America . . . The new FDA regulations will remove over 80 percent of the dietary supplements from the shelves of the neighborhood health food stores. The right of the American consumer to have freedom of choice in the foods he prefers to eat and the survival of the health-foods industry, a vital segment of the American free-enterprise system, lies in your hands.

gress [in opposition to the regulations] since the vitamin-mineral regulations were first proposed in January."

"Tens of thousands" was a huge understatement, as over 1 million Americans sent in letters and postcards—many of them yellow post-

---

PART 2 ■ FDA Raids and Abusive Tactics

Dr. Richard Passwater's interview with Frank Murray from 2005, entitled "FDA Injustices Against the Health Food Industry," discusses one particular example of an FDA raid, which took place in November 1988.

FDA made a raid on Traco Labs during November 1988. FDA claimed that black currant oil was an unsafe food additive when put into capsules. The FDA was claiming that any supplement other than vitamins and minerals with [an] established RDA would be a food additive and the manufacturer would have the burden of going through an extremely expensive FDA approval process to establish its safety. The odds were that the FDA would never grant the approval no matter what evidence was brought forth.

During the Traco raid, FDA seized two drums of black currant oil as well as a large quantity of filled capsules. I remember how attorney Robert Ullman dramatically convinced the judge that the FDA exceeded its regulatory authority. Bob first established that there were no safety concerns with black currant oil. Bob had placed several bottles of different oils on the table along with a few capsules. He asked the FDA's in-house expert witness if he had any objections if someone were to drink black currant oil or olive oil straight out of a bottle. The FDA witness responded with something like, "No one would do such a thing." Bob smiled; the trap had sprung. Bob opened a bottle and took a healthy drink.

He then asked the FDA lawyer to tell the judge what he was consuming. Was it food? Was it a food additive? His point was made to the judge. Then he swallowed a capsule filled with oil and looked at the judge and said, "And now it's a dangerous unproven food additive?"

The U.S. Court of Appeals ruled against the FDA on January 28, 1993, declaring that the agency's definition of food additive was too broad. The judge pointed out how, under the FDA's definition, even water could be considered a food additive when added to food. According to Dr. Passwater, the judge also criticized the FDA for its "Alice in Wonderland end run" around the law.

cards in order to draw attention—voicing their opposition to the proposed regulations. Along with these protests, the FDA faced numerous legal challenges brought forth by parties like the NNFA, represented by attorney Milton Bass. He ordered an injunction on the improperly issued regulations and submitted a blistering comment to the FDA in which he concluded, "The present law and regulations provide ample means for furnishing relevant information concerning vitamins and food supplements without imposing unnecessary, unreasonable and illegal prohibitions upon the consumer's freedom of choice in the selection of the foods he eats." The legal challenges posed by Bass, as well as New York attorney Robert Ullman, effectively prevented the "final" regulations from being rolled out and, therefore, enabled the Hosmer and Proxmire bills to pass. This legislation ensured the FDA's eventual defeat and American consumers' ultimate victory.

On September 24, 1974, the U.S. Senate passed the Hosmer-Proxmire Vitamin Bill by a vote of eighty-one to ten. Of the ten senators who voted in opposition, all of whom have since retired or passed away, eight were Democrats and two were Republicans. However, it took almost two years for the bill to be ironed out in the House and the Senate. It finally passed without dissent on April 12, 1976, and was signed into law as an attachment to the Heart and Lung Act, which was signed by President Gerald Ford on April 22, 1976.

The Hosmer-Proxmire Vitamin Bill laid the groundwork for DSHEA, which was enacted in 1994. "The National Nutritional Foods Association can take just pride for its role in this great accomplishment," wrote NNFA President Max Huberman and Milton Bass in July 1976, who hailed the bill as the "greatest victory for the health food industry and consumer rights ever achieved." And in a 2003 interview, Huberman said, "We were a force to be reckoned with."

THE ROAD TO DSHEA

In 1990, President George H.W. Bush signed the Nutrition Labeling and Education Act (NLEA), which was intended to improve nutritional information regarding products' health claims. The FDA was given the job of enforcing the act, but instead, they used its broad wording as an opportunity to over-regulate safe and beneficial nutritional products. The agency took the position that supplements with-

PART 3 ■ FDA Raids and Abusive Tactics

There were many raids in the years leading up to the passage of DSHEA. Here are just a few additional examples provided in Mike Adams' 2007 article for NaturalNews.com, "Tyranny in the USA."

El Cajon Pet Store Raid (1990). According to *Life Extension Magazine,* the FDA had been harassing Sissy Harrington-McGill, owner of Solid Gold Pet Foods in El Cajon, California, over labels on her holistic pet food products. In March 1990, an FDA agent seized products and literature from her store without a search warrant, and shut down her shop. Amazingly, Harrington-McGill would later be tried and convicted of violating the "Health Claims Law," which had never been passed by Congress and did not exist. After being indicted on July 12, 1990, she chose a jury trial, for which she was forced into leg irons, placed in a maximum-security federal prison for 179 days, and charged with a $10,000 fine. While in prison, Harrington-McGill suffered a near-fatal stroke.

Resolution: Harrington-McGill sued the U.S. Department of Justice and won her case in February 1992. As of 2007, she was planning to file a $25 million lawsuit against the FDA.

Highland Labs Raid (1990). Ken Scott, the owner of the Oregon-based vitamin company Highland Labs, offered to mail reprints of articles on the benefits of CoQ10 to customers who wanted to be more informed about the nutrient. In response, the FDA sent nine FDA agents, eleven U.S. marshals, and eight Oregon state police to Scott's business. The agents raided Highland Labs for eleven hours, confiscating countless items and threatening employees with violence if they tried to enter the office. Scott's daughter, who was miles away at the time, was illegally held under house arrest for twelve hours.

Resolution: On top of $250,000 in legal fees, Ken Scott was fined $5,000 and forced to plead guilty to selling unapproved new drugs. He was also forced to negotiate with prosecutors, serving five years probation for his "crime" of providing factual information about a beneficial nutrient.

NutriCology Raid (1991). Twelve armed FDA agents took part in the raid at NutriCology's offices and warehouse, after which the FDA took control of their bank accounts and shut down the company for two days. NutriCology was also charged with wire fraud, mail fraud, and selling unapproved drugs, misbranded drugs, and unsafe food additives.

Resolution: The FDA requested a preliminary injunction, but was denied by a federal judge on May 23, 1991, and then again by the 9th Circuit Court of Appeals in September 1991. The following year, in September 1992, the wire and mail fraud charges were eliminated, and the FDA's motion for summary judgment—judgment without a full trial—was denied.

out what it considered "defined nutritional value" were unapproved food additives. They then essentially went on an enforcement rampage.

According to Loren Israelsen, head of LDI Group and the Utah Natural Products Alliance based in Salt Lake City, the FDA was willing to go to "extreme lengths" to show that it was in control. "FDA was feeling really aggressive, like they could roll us whenever they wanted to," commented Israelsen in a 2004 article in *Natural Foods Merchandiser*. "[The agency] began using food additive provisions of the law as a tool to go after dietary supplements FDA did not like. This misuse of the law really ticked off a lot of people, me included." He also noted, "The FDA Commissioner at that time, David Kessler, had commissioned a panel to study the question, 'What should we do with supplements if we were to start afresh?' Initially, FDA refused to make the report public. Ultimately, under pressure they did, and it confirmed our worst fears." Israelsen added, "This is an example of the long fuse that burned up to 1992 when the first version of DSHEA called 'The Health Freedom Act' was introduced."

The Health Freedom Act, which was designed to protect the right of citizens to choose safe and effective dietary supplements, was introduced in the Senate by Senator Orrin Hatch, along with a similar bill in the House of Representatives sponsored by Representatives Bill Richardson of New Mexico and Elton Gallegly of California. The act proposed to expand the definition of dietary supplements to include herbs and other nutrients, thereby exempting supplement health claims from regulatory approval and prohibiting attempts to regulate supplements as drugs. In Israelsen's words, "The basic principle of the Health Freedom Act . . . was that supplements aren't food additives, they aren't drugs and they need to be defined."

Ultimately, however, the Health Freedom Act did not pass—but another bill did. The Dietary Supplement Act, which was added to the Prescription Drug User Fee Act of 1992, called for a one-year ban on dietary supplement health claims and nutrient content claims. Meanwhile, FDA raids continued, which only deepened the public's distrust of the agency.

The case that mobilized consumer opinion the most against the FDA was the Jonathan Wright case. Wright, a physician in Washington, had continued to prescribe the substance L-tryptophan to his patients, knowing that the U.S. had temporarily issued a ban on its sale as a dietary supplement. However, the medical use of L-tryptophan had not been explicitly banned.

On May 6, 1992, in what is today remembered as the Tahoma Clinic Raid, the FDA stormed Wright's clinic with armed sheriffs, who terrorized patients and seized vitamins, equipment, and medical records. According to Alex Schauss, "CFH discovered, after the FDA was forced by the state of Washington to explain the reason for the raid, that it was conducted in retaliation for Dr. Wright having filed a lawsuit against the FDA for restricting the availability of L-tryptophan as a dietary supplement."

The Tahoma Clinic raid raised concerns among American consumers. "People began to think, 'Wow, what are they [the FDA] prepared to do to stop us from taking vitamins?'" said Israelsen. This legitimate fear began to spread like wildfire across the country. Soon after, added Schauss, "Stores and clinics in other states reported similar raids. News of these events galvanized consumer support for passage of DSHEA."

There were also grassroots efforts to build support for DSHEA. To mobilize health food stores and consumers against the threat of raids, Joe Bassett (1932–2012) and the northwest region of the Natural Products Association (NPA), then the NNFA, expanded an early incarnation of what would later be called Citizens for Health (CFH). Other activists included Alex Schauss (as noted above), Jim Golick, Margaret Isely, Bonnie Minsky, Dr. Joan Priestley, Craig Winters, and others. There were also efforts made within the health industry; the American Botanical Council and the American Herbal Products Association (AHPA) were two particularly important forces. Moreover, industry champions such as Israelsen, Scott Bass (son of the late Milton Bass), Hal Drexler of Country Life, Jarrow Rogovin of Jarrow Formulas, and many others devoted considerable resources to the DSHEA battle.

Meanwhile, a dramatic public service ad (PSA) was made by a noted Los Angeles-based director/producer, Charles Abehsera. In the ad, federal agents fully equipped with Special Forces gear, including weapons and night vision gear, converge on Mel Gibson, who—in a now-famous cameo—holds up a supplement bottle and says, "Hey. Guys. Guys. It's only vitamins." Near the end of the ad, as Mel Gibson's character is being arrested, he says in desperation, "Vitamin C, you know, like in oranges?"

This call-to-action ad, which was funded by an industry task force that included Patrick Mooney of the California-based multivitamin company SuperNutrition and others, warned consumers that the federal government was "actually considering classifying most vitamins and other supplements as drugs. The FDA has already conducted raids on doctors' offices and health food stores. Could raids on individuals be next?" While the ad was definitely dramatic, the nightmarish scenario it portrayed was not far from reality at the time.

In May 1993, another dramatic yet effective tactic was used to educate consumers about the threats posed by the FDA. This "National Blackout Day," as it was called, was described by Bill Crawford of New Hope Natural Media, who was working at a health food store at the time:

> I vividly recall our putting on a "blackout" day. We got black mesh fabric and covered every product that would not be available for sale if DSHEA did not pass. It was nearly our entire supplement section! Products were available for sale but our staff was telling people why we had this restrictive covering . . . and signage . . . as well. Tables and chairs were set up for any customers who wanted to write a letter to Congress telling them how important access to dietary supplements was to them.

Although the Democrats had a majority in the House and Senate, there were signs that the party was in danger of losing seats in the 1994 elections. The Democrat leadership was not eager to look like the bad guys to the millions of Americans who supported the DSHEA.

Then, said Israelsen, "a miracle happened." Over the course of several hours, Senators Orrin Hatch, Ted Kennedy, and Tom Harkin, and Representatives Henry Waxman and John Dingell, were able to hammer out a compromise bill. "The bill never went through committee, and was never voted on, contrary to popular myth," Israelsen told *Natural Foods Merchandiser*. "It went from a zero, a nothing in the House, to being a bill flying through by unanimous consent in the middle of the night. I think the FDA thought this bill would never pass and when it did they couldn't believe it."

Although the story of how DSHEA was truly won is sometimes not told accurately, as Schauss has noted, "Those who made a difference know what contributions they made. They will always find satisfaction in having made a difference that influenced the course of history. Everyone made a difference. That's the real story that hasn't been told."

AFTER DSHEA: A TIMELINE

Following the passage of DSHEA, the health food industry was feeling good, and rightly so. It thus entered what might be called a laissez-faire period, marked by confidence on the one hand, but on the other, a low level of vigilance in regards to the FDA. In just a few years, the FDA resumed its anti-supplement, pro-pharma campaign, while at the same time trying to reclassify natural stages and conditions of life as "diseases" that could be treated with drugs. Other groups, such as the dietitian lobby, also stepped up their anti-supplement efforts (see the inset on page 85). By the end of the 1990s, the supplement industry was forced to wake from its slumber and, in the words of Shakespeare, "take arms against a sea of troubles." The timeline below marks key events in the ensuing struggle between the natural health industry and the FDA.

• **1996.** The White House Commission on Dietary Supplement Labels issues its report on future regulation of this product category. One year later, in 1997, the FDA publishes industry regulations for structure/function claims—fairly vague claims relating to general health rather than specific diseases—which, as per DSHEA, are allowed to appear on supplement packaging and marketing materials.

• **1997 to 1998.** In 1997, Congress adds a provision to the Food and Drug Modernization Act (FDAMA) that allows dietary supplements to make health claims. In addition, from the end of 1997 through early 1998, the Organic Trade Association (OTA) and Citizens for Health are able to stop the USDA from debasing the definition of "organic." Over a period of four months, nearly 300,000 communications are directed to the USDA in protest of the proposal, which is the largest number of comments the Department had ever received on any proposed regulation, according to the then Secretary of Agriculture, Daniel Glickman.

Back to its old tricks, in 1998, FDA inspectors arrive at the offices of a Texas-based stevia company to "witness destruction" of "offending" cookbooks featuring stevia and other literature. A video camera taping the aborted destruction, in combination with the intercession of Dr. Julian Whitaker and attorney Jim Turner, prevent the book burning.

• **1999.** The landmark case *Pearson v. Shalala* results in the FDA being

The Dietitian Lobby and Monopoly Control of Nutrition

To be fair, not all anti-supplement efforts have come from the FDA. Health professionals have also asserted their influence in the nutrition arena, particularly registered dietitians, or RDs. Registered dietitians are licensed by a private trade association, the Academy of Nutrition and Dietetics (AND), formerly known as the American Dietetic Association (ADA). They usually provide government-sanctioned dietary advice, such as the USDA Dietary Guidelines. This is in contrast to nutritionists, the other set of professionals that comprise approximately two-thirds of the nutrition community, who tend to take a very different approach to dietary advice by promoting optimal nutrition.

Despite the urgent need for more nutrition therapy and advice, nutritionists claim that the dietitian lobby has engaged in a campaign to monopolize nutrition advice through regulatory capture, such as state nutrition licensing laws and federal regulations. Dietitian licensing bills effectively make it a crime for non-RDs to give nutrition advice without a license. These laws also limit the number of nutrition advisors and professionals by essentially preventing them from practicing. In more than half of the U.S. states in which these one-sided licensure laws have passed, entire segments of practitioners—including naturopaths, herbalists, and many others—are often barred from providing advice.

Of course, regulatory capture of health professions is nothing new. But nutritionists say that the dietitian lobby's attempt is particularly egregious, as the scope of the dietetics and nutrition field is not a set of competencies unique to a particular type of healthcare provider, such as a nurse. In other words, "nutrition advice" is not a single profession, but a tool used by many different healthcare professionals, including medical doctors, naturopaths, acupuncturists, health coaches, and many more. Moreover, it does not involve substances that the law otherwise forbids the public to use, like prescription pharmaceuticals. Nutrition advice is based on a "substance" that is freely available to all and consumed every day: food. It is much more difficult, therefore, to reduce nutrition to a uniform regulatory scheme than it is for a discrete profession. It's like trying to license "exercise advice," which is a tool used by many kinds of health practitioners and therapists; it isn't the domain of a single profession.

According to the American Nutrition Association (ANA)—a non-profit organization representing nutritionists, health coaches, and other professionals who provide nutrition advice as part of their practices—the dietitian lobby is acting as a legislator, executive, judge, and jury in the following ways:

- It has attempted to include itself in federal regulations, so that only members of its professional trade group are permitted to be reimbursed for nutrition counseling.

- It has been fairly successful in getting state laws passed that are very similar to the North Carolina law that criminalizes the provision of nutrition advice—even when their own data shows a present shortage of nutrition professionals relative to the demand.

- Dietitian-friendly state laws make registered dietitians the dominant force on state licensing boards. These boards play a large role in determining who can and cannot obtain a license, first by drafting "rules" that spell out the details of licensure requirements—which are almost always the same as the dietitian group's requirements—and second, by acting as a gatekeeper for licensure applicants.

- The lobby encourages its members to file complaints against unlicensed practitioners to state licensing boards so that they can be prosecuted.

- Hearings and settlements that take place over the course of such prosecutions are conducted by or in close contact with the particular licensing board.

The sole beneficiaries of the dietitian lobby's drive for monopoly are its registered dietitians—and they are by no means the most highly qualified. The RD credential requires a bachelor's degree, whereas several other nutrition credentials require a master's degree or doctorate. What the dietitian lobby does have, though, is far greater financial resources. Still, ending the monopoly and ensuring protection for a diverse range of nutrition care providers is underway in states such as Illinois.

forced to allow qualified health claims. In March, consumer and industry advocates testify on Capitol Hill against the FDA's proposal to redefine disease to include life stages and normal discomforts, such as pregnancy, aging, menopause, and headache.

- **2005.** Despite the consumer backlash worldwide, Codex Draft Guidelines for Vitamin and Mineral Food Supplements are ratified. The European Food Supplements Directive (EFSD) also goes into effect.

- **2006.** Thanks in large part to the thousands of letters sent to legislators through a consumer-industry coalition, the "AER Bill" (the Dietary

Supplement and Nonprescription Drug Consumer Protection Act) passes in the U.S. House of Representatives at 3:06 AM on December 9, 2006. The new law adds to the extensive safety protections already in place for supplements, weakening the argument of critics claiming that supplement companies do not care about consumer safety.

- **2007.** The FDA issues a guidance on complementary and alternative medicine that could open the door to reclassifying common herbs, as well as fruit and vegetable juices, as "drugs," depending on their intended use. The action is successfully opposed by Citizens for Health and many other advocacy organizations.

- **2008.** On April 17, the FDA receives a Citizen Petition from a weight-loss drug manufacturer demanding that all weight-loss support claims be reclassified as disease claims. This move is strongly condemned by consumers and natural products industry organizations.

- **2009.** In March, the Food Safety Bill (S. 510) is introduced by Illinois Senator Richard Durbin. Many consumer advocates and industry experts point out that S. 510 and the House's version of the bill (H.R. 2749), which passed under suspended rules, do not address the root causes of the nation's food safety problems and, moreover, would hurt small growers and retailers. Fortunately, this misguided bill is scrapped.

- **2011.** On January 4, the Food Safety Modernization Act (FSMA) is signed into law, which, among other actions, forces the FDA to issue industry guidance as to when supplement ingredient manufacturers must submit New Dietary Ingredient (NDI) notifications to the agency. NDIs are dietary ingredients, such as vitamins, minerals, amino acids, herbs, or nutrient hybrids, that were not contained in dietary supplements marketed in the U.S. prior to the passage of DSHEA (October 15, 1994). Although this guidance had been mandated by DSHEA, it is not until July 1, 2011 that the FDA issues a draft guidance on NDIs. Many natural products organizations raise important objections to this guidance, including that it will stifle innovation, since the FDA tends to reject NDI submissions. Industry leaders also fear that the guidance will lead to unnecessary policies and procedures. In September 2011, Citizens for Health and Alliance for Natural Health launch a multi-pronged campaign to urge the FDA to revise or scrap the supplement-killing NDI Draft Guidance. The FDA later agreed to revise it.

Party Politics and Supplement Regulation

The fact that the majority of anti-supplement legislation comes from Democratic side of the aisle may lead one to wonder if Democrats downright hate supplements. The answer, of course, is no. There are many Democrats in Congress who happen to be stalwart champions of dietary supplements, including Iowa Senator Tom Harkin, as well as one of the greatest supplement-industry gladiators of all the time, Wisconsin Senator William Proximire from Wisconsin, one of the leaders behind the 1976 Hosmer-Proxmire Vitamin Bill. Still, political commentators have observed that the Democratic Party boasts at least a few more supplement foes in Congress than the Republican Party. Furthermore, Democrats have received (and continue to receive) a great deal of criticism from constituents and stakeholders for their weak and sometimes nonexistent response to the FDA's outrageous NDI Draft Guidance proposed in 2011. But do party labels really matter when it comes to dietary supplements?

Edward Long, PhD, Vice President of the lobbying firm Van Scoyoc Associates in Washington, DC, said in a 2008 interview that neither party is completely pro-supplement and pro-health freedom, and that different ideologies are represented in both the Democratic and Republican parties:

> There are two strains of Democrats. One is a populist strain, which goes back to the 1890s, the goo-goos, the good government people who believe that American citizens need to be protected by government in every possible way and to be told what to do. It's from this camp that a few of dietary supplements' greatest critics have emerged. Then there's the most liberal, anarchistic side of the Democratic Party that goes back to the 1960s and 1970s, which holds that mainstream medicine doesn't really work. It's out of this strain that we have found a few of dietary supplements' greatest advocates.

As for the Republicans, according to Long, while there is a sizeable subset of the Republican Party that is opposed to government regulation and over-regulation, "there's another strain that believes that, in certain cases, we need more regulation."

Unfortunately, however, the "goo-goos" from the Democratic Party have been consistently proposing, co-sponsoring, and advocating the worst pieces of anti-supplement legislation since the bipartisan passage of DSHEA in 1994. One of the most recent examples is Senator Durbin's Amendment 2127, which was defeated by a vote of seventy-seven to twenty, and which would have made it extremely difficult to register dietary supplements, even those that have already been deemed safe. The amendment also would have made supplement labeling submission requirements resemble the kind of drug-like regulations that are being implemented in Canada and Europe today (see page 119).

Looking back to 2011, Senator Patrick Leahy's Food Safety and Accountability Act (S. 216, originally introduced as S. 3767), which essentially allows the FDA to criminalize nearly any food or food supplement based on labeling or unintentional contamination, was a fully Democrat-sponsored bill. It passed the Senate in April 2011 and is still awaiting a vote in the House as of the publication of this book. Moreover, two much-despised House bills from 2009, Rosa DeLauro's Food Safety Modernization Act lookalike and Jim Costa's so-called food safety legislation (which only boosts the power of the FDA), were largely supported by Democrats. The former was a 100-percent Democratic-sponsored bill, and 66 percent of Democrats backed the latter.

Of course, not all anti-supplement legislation originates on the "donkey" side of the aisle. In 2010, Republican Senator John McCain introduced the widely vilified Dietary Supplement Safety Act of 2010 (S. 3002), which he was forced to withdraw due to massive grassroots opposition.

It's important to remember that although most, if not all, anti-supplement bills carry the word "safety" in their titles, they do not truly advance consumer safety. Rather, these bills reduce consumer access to high-quality, high-potency, and innovative supplements. They are, therefore, *anti*-safety, or at least anti-health. In order to fully understand the significance, intention, and potential consequences of health legislation in Congress, it's important to look beyond the bill title.

Today, together with the outreach efforts of fellow health freedom groups and the natural products industry, advocates for health freedom have been successful in their efforts to get the FDA to go back to the drawing board regarding the NDI Draft Guidance. According to *Natural Products INSIDER*, "After close to a year of industry outcry, FDA apparently will issue a revised draft guidance on the topic of new dietary ingredients (NDIs)."

What Are ODIs and NDIs?

Ever since DSHEA was passed, the subject of dietary ingredients was a gray area. Nevertheless, it was universally accepted that the natural products industry's master lists of herbal ingredients, for example, were safe, having been published in the authoritative *Herbs of Commerce,* as well as submitted to the FDA without question or objection for over sixteen years.

DSHEA set a clear distinction between "old" and "new" dietary ingredients for supplements. The law officially regarded *old dietary ingredients* (ODIs) as nutritional ingredients (nutrients and herbal extracts) that were sold prior to 1994. ODIs were considered to be "grandfathered in" and "generally recognized as safe," so supplement ingredient manufacturers did not have to worry about reporting food-based supplements or ingredients that had always been in the food supply.

New dietary ingredients (NDIs), on the other hand, were defined as completely new compounds, often hybrids of nutrients, never before seen in nature in exactly that form. To consider these ingredients "new," however, was strange, since many safe nutrients are often combined with other safe natural substances in order to enhance the absorption of a particular mineral or vitamin. How could these benign compounds be classified as "new" when compared, for example, to products of genetically engineered bacterial fermentation?

Some supplement companies were advised by legal experts against submitting NDI notifications, since the ingredients in question were already technically considered safe and, therefore, were exempt from the new requirements. On top of that, the FDA was rejecting so many NDI submissions—on seemingly arbitrary and capricious grounds—that companies, understandably, began to view the NDI process as an impenetrable obstacle to approval.

Fortunately, as of 2013, the FDA is in the process of revising their requirements for NDIs thanks to the efforts of health freedom advocates, organizations, and natural products companies.

WHAT YOU CAN DO

One of the best ways to ensure a better playing field for dietary supplements, as well as health freedom in general, is to support promising bills, oppose anti-health freedom bills, and be more aware of present and future health-related issues. Below are some facts and suggestions that may be helpful for deciding which issues to support and which to oppose.

1. Spiked supplements are not dietary supplements. So-called "spiked" supplements—products intentionally adulterated with designer anabolic steroids, stimulants, or prescription drugs—are not dietary supplements, but rather illegal or unapproved drugs posing as supplements. They should be immediately referred to the U.S. Drug Enforcement Administration (DEA) so that appropriate action can be taken.

Twenty Years After DSHEA: A Reflection

What do experts think about the passage of DSHEA? I asked Jonathan Emord, a Constitutional scholar and attorney, his thoughts on the landmark legislation, now nearly twenty years since it was signed into law. Here is what he had to say:

For decades, FDA manipulated the definition of dietary supplements. In 1994, Congress enacted DSHEA following intense public debate concerning the importance of dietary supplements in promoting health, the need for consumers to have access to current and accurate information about supplements, and controversy over the FDA's actions to remove dietary supplements from the market and suppress speech concerning supplements. Some view the DSHEA as perfect. It is far from that. When former Hatch aide Patricia Knight assembled lawyers, including me, in a room to evaluate DSHEA's provisions and recommend changes, I objected to several of the bill's provisions. For example, I thought the provisions requiring the filing of notice of structure/function claims [were] fraught with danger, because I knew that sooner or later, FDA would use the notice filing requirement as a means to challenge the claims. I also thought the third-party literature provision unwise because the definitional requirements of that provision, together with FDA's intended use doctrine, could defeat its intended meaning. In general, we preferred removing jurisdiction of the FDA over problem areas, rather than attempting to legislate avenues for regulation in those areas. Our objections fell on deaf ears, but our predictions of agency mischief in interpreting DSHEA's provisions proved prophetic.

Recommendation: SUPPORT the Anabolic Steroid Control Act (S. 3431) sponsored by Senator Sheldon Whitehouse (D-RI).

2. In general, oppose bills introduced by Senator Richard Durbin. Durbin is notoriously anti-supplements, so be wary of any bill he brings to the floor, especially those with the word "safety" in the title. A perfect example is the Dietary Supplement Labeling Act (S. 1310). According to the National Health Federation (NHF), "Senator Durbin is using this bill as his vehicle for other purposes, mainly to strangle the supplement industry and dry up supply to consumers. [The bill's] real purpose is to establish expensive, drug-like FDA approval requirements for proving the safety of [already safe] supplements."

Recommendation: OPPOSE the Dietary Supplement Labeling Act sponsored by Senator Richard Durbin (D-IL).

3. Support bills endorsed by Citizens for Health, the National Health Federation, and the Alliance for Natural Health. The Dietary Supplement Protection Act (H.R. 3380) is just one example. This bill would give pre-approved "grandfather" status to all dietary supplement ingredients introduced up through 2007. If passed, manufacturers of these nutritional ingredients won't be forced to jump through ridiculous or onerous hoops if the FDA has its way with any version of the NDI Draft Guidance. As NHF's Scott Tips rightly notes, while the bill is "not a panacea for all of the problems found in the NDI Draft Guidance," it is a "politically expedient 'salami slice for freedom' that will take care of our FDA problem for now."

Recommendation: SUPPORT the Dietary Supplement Protection Act (DSPA), or H.R. 3380, sponsored by Representative Dan Burton (R-IN).

4. Consumers should have access to the nutrient P5P. The FDA is considering a petition filed by the U.S. subsidiary of a Canadian pharmaceutical company, Medicure, Inc. According to the Alliance for Natural Health (ANH), Medicure is requesting a ban on dietary supplements that contain pyridoxal 5'-phosphate (P5P), the bioactive, natural form of vitamin B6, so that they can sell it as a drug. A spokesperson for the ANH remarked, "Last time we checked, FDA's mission was to protect and advance the public health. So if P5P already exists in nature [and] we can't live without it, and [if it] has a multiplicity of positive health effects, for example, on carpal tunnel, schizophrenia, and cancer, then how does banning P5P further either of the FDA's goals?" The passage of DSPA will prevent the FDA and Medicure from making P5P readily available to the public.

Recommendation: SUPPORT the Dietary Supplement Protection Act (DSPA), or H. R. 3380.

CONCLUSION:
WHERE DO WE GO FROM HERE?

So far, this book has covered the origins of the natural health and health foods movement, the transformation of the food supply, and the major political battles industry leaders have fought to attain—and maintain—consumer access to beneficial dietary supplements. Now, looking forward, what are the biggest health threats?

When it comes to supplements, "we are up against two main antagonists," opined Jarrow Rogovin, president of the nutritional supplement company Jarrow Formulas. He identified these as the "institutionalized and ingrained" attitude of the FDA, and the "left-wing statists who want minute government control of everything and are averse to individual decision-making."

As Roy Upton has observed, "We live in a country where we can own and use weapons, smoke cigarettes that kill more than 400,000 Americans annually, drink alcohol, which kills approximately 75,000 Americans annually, and supplements can't legally be used to treat disease; go figure!"

In addition to the natural health industry's domestic struggles, there are also international challenges to our health freedom thanks to a globalized food economy and industry. International guidelines, which are formally known as the United Nations FAO/WHO Codex Alimentarius, and the difficulties they pose for the supplement industry—and therefore, your health—are examined in the next chapter.

4

The Global Fix

Food Insecurity,
Supplement Regulation, and Codex

*"If we can imagine food freedom and work to make it real in
our everyday lives, we will have challenged food dictatorship."*

—VANDANA SHIVA, *STOLEN HARVEST,* 2000

Global trade dates back to some of the world's oldest civilizations, and served as the vehicle for cultural, religious, and artistic exchanges on the one hand, and monopolies, exploitation, oppression, and war on the other. Trade also created concerns about low-quality food and commodities. Early historical records show that even in ancient times, many societies had codes and laws in place to protect consumers from dishonest practices in the sale of food. Egyptian scrolls set out the rules for "food labeling," and in ancient Greece, beer and wine was inspected for purity. The Romans also had a well-organized food-control system that protected citizens from fraud and bad produce. And during the Middle Ages, laws were passed to regulate the quality and safety of eggs, cheese, beer, wine, and bread in Europe.

Today, food safety and consumer protection are still concerns, as the global trade of food, food additives, agricultural chemicals, and pharmaceutical drugs has grown to unparalleled levels. Globalization of the food industry and trade system has led to the development of beneficial, world-recognized standards, which has enhanced food safety around the world. At the same time, however, globalization has brought international food-safety disasters, such as the 1971 poison grain disaster in Iraq, which killed over 650 people, and the 1981 rape-seed disaster in Spain, which claimed over 600 lives. More recently, there has been an increased incidence of mad cow disease, as well as contamination due to bacteria like salmonella and E. coli. The rise in these kinds of catastrophes has made it clear that the world is in dire need of higher standards for food safety.

Unfortunately, instead of implementing an effective strategy for dealing with food safety issues, the world has taken a politically palatable approach marked by agreement with international food safety guidelines known as Codex Alimentarius (Latin for "food code"). These guidelines are proposed by members of the Codex Alimentarius Commission (CAC), a global body established by the World Health Organization (WHO) and Food and Agriculture Organization (FAO) to make recommendations on issues related food standards and trade practices. While Codex guidelines can be useful for developing countries that lack their own food safety standards, they often inhibit manufacturers and consumers in countries that have more liberal laws, especially in terms of supplement regulation. This chapter outlines major conflicts that have emerged over trade and food standards as a result of globalization and Codex guidelines.

THE RISE OF GLOBALISM

The early twentieth century was a turbulent time, both in the United States and abroad. Less than thirty years after the virulent influenza pandemic of 1890, the U.S. was dealt another blow known as the Great Pandemic, or Spanish Flu. In three waves between 1918 and 1919, the Flu claimed a total of over 675,000 American lives. Recent estimates place global mortality from the pandemic at anywhere from 30 to 50 million deaths.

Yet, it wasn't until 1932 when, according to contemporary historian William Manchester, America truly hit "rock bottom." Reeling from the stock market crash of 1929, which served as the catalyst for the Great Depression, the U.S. faced rising unemployment (at 1 million and increasing), about half a million foreclosed farms, more than 5,000 failed banks, and approximately 86,000 bankrupt businesses. Lacking safety nets like unemployment insurance, Medicare, and Social Security, people had few, if any, places to turn.

According to Sally Denton in *The Plots Against the President* (2012), in a desperate effort to drive up prices, farmers killed their livestock and burned their fields. A telling contemporary report stated that Iowa farmers "dump their milk trying to get the price up to where they can keep producing milk so babies won't go hungry." Historian Jean Edward Smith, author of *FDR*, noted, "In Iowa, a bushel of corn was worth less than a package of chewing gum. In the South, thousands of acres of fine, long-staple cotton stood in the field unpicked, the cost of ginning exceeding any possible return." In cities, panhandlers gathered on corners, and "children suffering from malnutrition sold pathetic scraps of food and clothes. People combed garbage dumps for usable items, often fighting over caches of kindling . . . Boxcar hoboes and disheveled migrant children haunted the newsreels."

The effects of the Great Depression were also felt in Europe, which was still struggling to recover and rebuild in the wake of World War I. Even with aid from the United States—which had shipped over 6 million tons of food commodities to Europe between 1919 and 1926—England experienced a severe economic depression, known there as the Great Slump. The effects on Britain's industrial areas were instantaneous and severe. As the demand for British products sharply declined, the value of exports dropped by 50 percent, the unemployment rate doubled, and the national income average fell. The government also lost money, faced with the task of providing assistance to the rising number of jobless and destitute people. According to a government report from the mid-1930s, approximately 25 percent of the UK's population were forced to follow a subsistence diet, and child malnutrition was widespread, leading to scurvy, rickets, and tuberculosis.

In *World Food Security*, D. John Shaw noted that in the early 1930s, Yugoslavia proposed that the Health Division of the League of Nations, the intergovernmental organization created after World War I, "disseminate information about the food position in representative countries of the world" to acknowledge the importance of food to overall health. Eventually, the League of Nations recognized the fact that increasing food production to meet the needs of the global population would boost both agriculture and industry, bringing "the needed expansion of the world economy through what was described as 'the marriage of health and agriculture.'"

In an effort to stem the tide in the United States, President Franklin D. Roosevelt, who took office on March 4, 1933, enacted the New Deal, a series of economic programs rolled out between 1933 and 1936. This suite of programs focused on what historians call the "3 Rs": relief for the unemployed and poor; recovery of the economy to normal levels; and reform of the financial system to prevent a repeat depression. One particularly important piece of legislation that was passed is the Agricultural Adjustment Act of 1933, which—among other provisions—provided subsidies to farmers via the Grain Stabilization Board. Also established was the Commodity Credit Corporation (CCC), an entity owned and operated by the U.S. government intended to protect and stabilize farm income and prices. Initially, it was closely affiliated with the Reconstruction Finance Corporation, but was transferred to the USDA in July 1939. The CCC proved to be a huge boost to the economy, making FDR's first term one of the fastest period of gross domestic product (GDP) growth in U.S. history.

At the same time, Roosevelt took steps to build international relationships. When France and England came under siege by Germany in 1940, for example, Roosevelt provided as much aid as possible short of actual military involvement. He also focused on the planning of the United Nations, which he hoped would replace the League of Nations and serve as a strong, cooperative global body for resolving international difficulties, including the problems of hunger and malnutrition. These problems, which had been greatly exacerbated by the war, were the subject of the UN Conference on Food and Agriculture, which convened in May 1943 in Hot Springs, Virginia.

According to the FAO, the Hot Springs conference set up an interim commission focused on food and agriculture to "help governments consider the formulation and adoption of similar international standards of . . . purity for all foods." This commission made wide-ranging recommendations on nutrition and standards for the basic composition of foods, as well as the containers, additives, pesticides, fertilizers, and other materials used in food production and distribution. It also urged governments to take steps to "ensure that producers and consumers are adequately protected against trade malpractices and against exploitation in the purchase and sale of food," according to the journal *AgBioForum*. Finally, leaders at the Conference pointed out the need for a bigger, more accessible food supply in order to both reduce

Milestones in the Development of Codex

- **1945.** The Food and Agriculture Organization (FAO) is founded, with responsibilities "covering nutrition and associated food standards."

- **1948.** The World Health Organization (WHO) is established, with responsibilities "covering human health and, in particular, a mandate to establish food standards."

- **1950.** Joint FAO/WHO meetings begin on nutrition, food additives, and related areas.

- **1953.** WHO's highest governing body, the World Health Assembly, announces that the "widening use of chemicals in the food industry presents a new public health problem that needs attention."

- **1960.** The first FAO Regional Conference for Europe endorses the "desirability of international—as distinct from regional—agreement on minimum food standards and invites the Organization's Director-General to submit proposals for a joint FAO/WHO" program on food standards to the FAO.

- **1961.** The Council of the Codex Alimentarius Europaeus adopts a resolution proposing that its work on food standards be taken over by FAO and WHO. With the support of WHO, the Economic Commission for Europe (ECE), the Organization for Economic Cooperation and Development (OECD), and the Council of the Codex Alimentarius Europaeus, the FAO Conference establishes Codex Alimentarius and resolves to create an international food standards program. They also decide to set up the Codex Alimentarius Commission and request an early endorsement by WHO of a joint FAO/WHO food standards program.

- **1962.** The Joint FAO/WHO Food Standards Conference asks the Codex Commission to implement the Joint FAO/WHO Food Standards Program.

- **1963.** The World Health Assembly approves establishment of the Joint FAO/WHO Food Standards Program and adopts the statutes of the Codex Alimentarius Commission.

Source: "Understanding Codex Alimentarius." FAO/WHO, 1999.

and prevent the widespread problem of malnutrition. Recommendations from the UN Conference directly led to the creation of the FAO in October 1945 and the World Health Organization (WHO) in 1948.

In May 1963, with the devastation and food insecurity of World War II still fresh in the world's memory, the WHO's decision-making body, the World Health Assembly, approved the establishment of the Joint FAO/WHO Food Standards Program. The governing body formed to implement this program was the Codex Alimentarius Commission (CAC), which was dedicated to "protecting the health of consumers and facilitating trade in foods" by defining and enforcing the standards of the Codex Alimentarius. As you will see, the impact of the Codex Alimentarius on health freedom has made it a source of controversy, as well as misinformation and confusion.

FOOD (IN)SECURITY TODAY

Despite international efforts to curb problems like world hunger and effectively regulate the food supply, food insecurity continues today, due in large part to globalization itself. At the first international food conference in 1974, Henry Kissinger, the U.S. Secretary of State, promised that by 1984, no man, woman, or child would go hungry. Of course, at the time, the planet was inhabited by 4 billion people and the world grain harvest per capita was growing. Today, the world population is nearly 7 billion, and since 1984—Kissinger's projected end-of-hunger milestone—the rate of grain-yield increase has been steadily falling. According to John Robbins, we have every reason to believe that "this decline will accelerate in coming years as aquifiers [underground layers of water-bearing rock] are depleted and water for irrigation becomes increasingly scarce."

While grain yields per acre have been increasing, as noted, the *rate* of increase has been slowing since the days of the Green Revolution of the 1970s. Most of the benefits of irrigation, machinery, fertilizer, and plant breeding have already been realized. In fact, the production of grain per acre is close to the maximum amount obtainable through photosynthesis. According to the Worldwatch Institute, there are several reasons for this, including climate change, deforestation, land degradation, decreasing oil and water supplies, animal extinction, the destruction of ecosystems, and the environmental demands caused by meat-rich diets in developed countries. Lying at the center of these problems is the exploitation of the planet's resources, as well as unprecedented population growth. Experts say that keeping up with this rate of growth will require more food to be produced over the next fifty years than has been produced over the past 10,000 years. Currently, at least 1.2 billion people across the globe don't get enough to eat and are suffering from hunger, while an additional 2 to 3.5 billion suffer from vitamin and mineral deficiency. These alarming statistics reveal not only the effects of globalization on the world food supply, but also the seemingly illogical relationship between increased food and output and the continued prevalence of hunger and malnutrition. According to a 2003 report from what was then known as the American Dietetic Association (ADA):

> Food insecurity was once viewed as a problem of inadequate food production, and emphasis was placed on increasing national food supplies to deal with hunger. Such an approach is necessary, but insufficient. Hunger exists today, even after a half century during which world food output nearly tripled.

The reason for this may lie in globalization itself, which has essentially destroyed sustainable food systems. In *Stolen Harvest* (2000), Vandana Shiva wrote, "Globalization has created the McDonaldization of world food. . . . It attempts to create a uniform food culture of hamburgers." She also pointed to the consequences of this "uniform food culture" on the environment and the food supply:

> For every pound of red meat, poultry, eggs, and milk produced, farm fields lose about five pounds of irreplaceable top soil. The water necessary for meat breeding comes to about 190 gallons per animal per day, or 10 times what a normal Indian family is supposed to use in one day, if it gets water at all.

Another problem related to this issue is that some of the available national data on food supplies masks regional differences. For example, while China and Thailand have pledged to reduce hunger, high rates of under-nutrition still persist in certain regions. In fact, according to the ADA report, "nearly 80% of all malnourished children in the developing world live in countries that report *food surpluses*" (emphasis mine). There are many ways to approach this problem, but when it comes to food security, most authorities point to the importance of people having control over land and access to credit, such as microcredit—small loans typically given to impoverished individuals.

Furthermore, as Dr. H. Curtis Wood points out in *Overfed But Undernourished,* although hunger and malnutrition are widespread problems, the notion of so-called "overnutrition" deceives the industrialized world into thinking that because there is sufficient food for all, (1) everybody gets it, and (2) it is of high nutritional value, which is not at all the case. *Overnutrition* is more properly called *overconsumption,* as it describes the intake of food and nutrients to the point where it adversely affects your health. The prevalence of this condition in developed countries is due to the twentieth century's uneven prosperity wave of food abundance and nutrient scarcity, which, as Gary Gardner and Brian Halweil explained in *Underfed and Overfed,* swept up "millions . . . to new diets that were often bountiful but nutritionally deficient."

In addition to hunger, malnutrition, and damage to the environment, today's globalized food culture and food economy has another hidden cost: food contamination. In 2011, physicists at the University of Notre Dame, Mária Ercsey-Ravasz and Zoltán Toroczkai, in collaboration with food science experts József Baranyi and Zoltán Lakner, conducted an analysis of the international food-trade network that showed its vulnerability to the fast spread of contaminants. They also observed a correlation between known outbreaks of food poisoning and the centrality of countries in the international agro-food trade network (IFTN), a core group of seven nations that trade food products with over 77 percent of countries in the world:

> Since any two countries in the IFTN have only two degrees of separation on the network, the IFTN is capable of spreading a food-borne contaminant very efficiently. . . . It also tends to mask the contaminant's origins once the system is compromised, since so many network paths run through the central nodes.

In other words, the handful of countries that trade with over three-quarters of the world, by the very breadth and depth of their reach in the network, can very easily and rapidly spread contamination throughout the globe with the foodstuffs they trade.

By 2030, food demand is expected to increase by 50 percent. Since the 1960s, global food transport has been increasing at an exponential rate—more quickly than food production itself. As the system grows, so does pressure on regulation and surveillance organizations to track contaminants and prevent deadly outbreaks, such as those that occurred in 2011 in the U.S. (*Listeria monocytogenes*) and Germany (*Escherichia coli*). While the researchers didn't go so far as to predict an increase in food poisoning cases, the report predicted delays in determining the sources of contamination and, therefore, recommended identifying and correcting the trade network's vulnerabilities.

Today, the Codex Alimentarius Commission, or simply "Codex," continues to shamble along in its efforts to standardize and globalize international food, food trade, and food purity standards and guidelines. These efforts have been a source of controversy and debate, as they included an attempt to impose pharmaceutical-like regulations on nutritional supplements in 2004. In response, the FDA predicted that the U.S. would eventually need to dumb down, or "harmonize" (see the inset on page 105) its own supplement regulations in keeping with the international standards. As you will see, this has done little to reassure American consumers, and has only served to mobilize the natural health industry.

CODEX, EUROPE, AND THE UNITED STATES

Since its inception, there has been much debate, information, and misinformation surrounding Codex because of how it has impacted health freedom. While Codex has demonstrated a distrust of food supplements, it has implemented liberal policies towards synthetic—and potentially harmful—food additives. As mentioned earlier, the stated mission of the Codex Alimentarius Commission, which is today based in Rome, Italy, is to "protect the health of consumers" and to "ensure fair practices in the international food trade" by developing food standards, guidelines, and related texts, such as codes of practice. Consisting of 185 member countries plus the European Union (which itself is made up of 27 member nations), Codex is responsible for promoting coordination of all food standards work undertaken by international governmental and non-governmental organizations (NGOs).

The Secretary of the Codex Alimentarius Commission is a senior FAO official who serves as the Chief of the Joint FAO/WHO Food Standards Programs, and is assisted by the Commission's Secretariat, which is comprised of six full-time officials based at the FAO Headquarters. Subsidiary Codex Committees, such as the Committee on Fats and Oils, are financially maintained and operated by governments of member nations, with oversight from the Secretariat. There are also Coordinating Committees—for example, the Coordinating Committee for Latin America and the Caribbean, or CCLAC—which are larger entities by which entire global regions or groups of countries coordinate and develop food standards activities for their own particular regions. There may be as many as twenty international Codex committee meetings in any twelve-month period. NGOs, which may represent consumers or a certain industry, are allowed to address the Commission, but they do not vote on any decisions pertaining to standards and guidelines.

The U.S. Codex Office in the USDA's Food Safety and Inspection Service houses and provides staff support for the United States representatives to the Codex Commission. The staff of the U.S. Codex Office works closely with the U.S. delegates to various Codex Commission committees, as well as government agencies, NGOs, members of Congress, and the general public. The Codex Office also receives resource support from the FDA, which acts as the food safety consultant for U.S. representatives to Codex.

In *Understanding the Codex Alimentarius* (1999), the Commission lists over 4,000 standards, guidelines, and codes that have been promulgated in ten subject areas: commodities, codes of practice, food labeling, food hygiene, food safety risk assessment, contaminants in foods, maximum limits for pesticide residents, maximum limits for veterinary drugs in foods, food additives provisions, and finally, sampling, analysis, inspection, and certification procedures. Although Codex has created some problems (see the insets on page 105 and 107), according to John R. Lupien in a 2000 issue of *AgBioForum:*

> In practice, over the past 40 years Codex has served as a very effective mechanism for obtaining consensus among Codex member

countries on a wide range of food standards for individual food products, food labeling, recommendations on pesticide residue food additive and food contaminant levels, codes of hygienic practice, and other recommendations.

The Cost of "Trade Friendly" Supplements

Although one of the primary goals of Codex is to "ensure fair practice in food trade," their success in this area is questionable. While at first blush "free trade" may seem like a pro-liberty or pro-freedom concept, in the case of supplements, trade is only "free" if it's also Codex-friendly. In other words, free trade comes at a cost; specifically, supplements made by U.S. companies must be drastically "dumbed down" in order to comply with Codex standards, which set very low maximum permitted levels of basic vitamins and minerals. In fact, these levels are even lower than the U.S. government-established RDAs, which are already very low. The maximum permitted level of vitamin D, for instance, is 5 micrograms (mcg), whereas the RDA is 15 to 20 mcg for adult men.

The type of trade being promoted by Codex hurts global consumers because it restricts access to effective nutritional supplements. Innovative American supplement manufacturers are also hurt, since their high-potency, high-quality products are encountering major trade barriers that masquerade as "safety standards." While indirectly forcing supplement makers to "dumb down" the ingredients in their products may not have been its original intention, this is the direction in which the Codex Commission is headed thanks to its misguided risk-assessment framework and binding international treaties. The U.S. Codex Delegation will likely follow in its footsteps with the growing influence of corporations and Big Agriculture- and Big Pharma-friendly trade associations.

Given the strong safety record of nutritional supplements—which are derived from a historically nutrient-dense world diet that has been 10,000 years in the making—upper-safe levels of ingredients should be implemented and regarded the same way as are RDAs in the United States. RDAs, which must be listed by the manufacturer, serve as recommendations for consumers. They are not mandated potency limits signed off on by the government, nor are they trade barriers that block consumer access to health-optimizing levels of nutrients.

But how successful has Codex been in cooperating with the national laws of its member countries, such as the much debated Food Supplements Directive of the European Union, the U.S. Dietary Supplement Health and Education Act (DSHEA), and FDA standards and regulations?

As already mentioned, the FDA serves as the consultant to U.S. Codex representatives on matters regarding food safety and quality, which includes supplements. The agency has often sided with the European Union (EU)—which has twenty-seven Codex votes—in efforts to move the whole world towards the EU's position that essential nutrients can be obtained from food alone, that supplements are dangerous in high potencies, that vitamins and minerals should be subject to the same risk assessment as dangerous chemicals and additives, and that supplement use should be minimized and restricted. The Codex has already adopted this position with support from the international supplement industry, as well as a few large American and multinational corporations that manufacture low-quality supplements using cheap ingredients.

Although the FDA has a similar attitude to that of the European Union when it comes to supplements, its actual policies differ. The official view of European regulators is that individuals can get all the nutrients they need from food. They also have "positive" and "negative" lists of supplements to differentiate between those that have been proven safe and effective—and thus can be sold—and those that cannot be sold. The United States, on the other hand, has no such lists, and official FDA policy does not hold that all necessary nutrients are present in food sources. Moreover, nutrients are presumed safe unless the FDA proves them to be harmful.

These policies were established by DSHEA, which, as explained in Chapter Three, was passed in October 1994 and legitimized the view that dietary supplements can complement a daily diet and provide health benefits. It also acknowledged that there may be a positive relationship between sound dietary practice and good health, as well as a connection between supplement use, disease prevention, and reduced healthcare expenses. Addressing the concerns of supplement consumers and manufacturers, DSHEA helped to ensure that safe and appropriately labeled supplement products would be made available to those who wanted to use them. DSHEA also defined dietary supplements and dietary ingredients, established a new framework for assuring safety, and outlined guidelines for literature displayed where supplements are sold. The law also provided for use of claims and nutritional support statements, required ingredient and nutrition labeling, and granted authority to the FDA to set good manufacturing practice (GMP) regulations. In addition, DSHEA required the creation of an executive-level Commission on Dietary Supplements and an Office of Dietary Supplements within the National Institutes of Health (NIH). These provisions served as positive recognition of supplement producers and consumers, and provided protection against the loss of access to these products. The FDA, however, has disagreed with DSHEA from the beginning, and continues to try to undermine it in every way.

The relationships between DSHEA and Codex, DSHEA and the EU Food Supplement Directive, and Codex and the Directive, are tangential. Here's how it works: Each country (or member state in the Codex Commission) has its own food rules, laws, regulations, and accepted practices. In order to promote international trade, Codex works to get its 185 member countries to adopt proposed guidelines and standards via a formal multistep process that often takes years to complete, if it is completed at all. Although it's not mandatory for member countries

Codex and Big Industry

Along with other nations, the United States has used a pro-big industry strategy when it comes to special interests. For example, when high-fructose corn syrup, which has been linked to obesity and other epidemics, was first proposed as a food additive, the FDA was reluctant to grant approval. However, corn growers approached Codex via trade associations and gained a Codex standard allowing its use as an additive. Lobbyists for the corn industry then re-approached the FDA and used Codex's "blessing" as ammunition to convince the agency to approve high-fructose corn syrup as well. Their argument can more or less be summed up as, "If Codex, the international voice of food standards, has adopted high-fructose corn syrup, it must be good." The FDA acquiesced, harmonizing its policies—in other words, overriding its own rules—with the international standard. Since then, high-fructose corn syrup has become ubiquitous in the food supply, and Americans, especially children, have become less healthy.

to adopt Codex guidelines, doing so is one way to ensure that they do not violate trade rules established by the World Trade Organization.

Still, there are some problems with this system, as Jim Turner, the chair of the non-profit health advocacy group Citizens for Health, has pointed out. "Together these laws, regulations and guidelines represent a complex matrix mainly navigable by well-heeled corporations and trade associations," he said. "It is well nigh impenetrable by underfunded individuals, citizens groups, and anyone else who puts health and well-being ahead of market efficiency and money." No case has better illustrated this interconnected, complicated, and nearly impenetrable relationship than the controversy surrounding the Codex's Guidelines for Vitamin and Mineral Food Supplements.

THE SUPPLEMENT CONTROVERSY

The supplement controversy involving Codex, Europe, and the U.S. began in 1996, when the German delegation to Codex Commission issued a proposal stating that no herb, vitamin, or mineral should be sold for preventive or therapeutic reasons, and that supplements should be classified as drugs, not foods. The proposal set off massive global outrage among supplement producers and consumers, whose protests halted its implementation.

Between 1996 and 2005, Codex committees worked to develop what became the official Codex Guidelines for Vitamin and Food Supplements, which were adopted in Rome on July 4, 2005. While the Guidelines do not ban any supplements outright, they do subject them to labeling and packaging requirements, set criteria for establishing maximum and minimum dosage levels, and require that safety and efficacy be considered when setting ingredients sources. The Guidelines also maintain that consumers can get the nutrients they need from food.

Although more restrictive than some national supplement laws like DSHEA, many supplement manufacturer organizations generally support the Guidelines. The International Alliance of Dietary/Food Supplement Associations (IADSA), whose member associations include manufacturers of the vast majority of supplements worldwide, initially favored the Guidelines because they reversed much of the draconian proposal issued by Germany in 1996. For example, the Codex

Health Organizations Comment on Codex

While most health advocacy groups agree that individuals should be able to assess their own unique nutritional needs and buy supplements of their choosing, many of them take slightly different approaches to this issue. Opinions expressed by three major health organizations are presented below.

Alliance for Natural Health (ANH). The ANH runs a campaign focused on reversing Codex policies that set very low maximum daily doses for dietary supplements, use flawed risk assessment methods, categorize therapeutic nutrients as drugs, and establish requirements for clinical trials that are too expensive for small companies. The campaign also opposes the setting of unnecessarily low Nutrient Reference Values, which seriously understate requirements for long-term optimum health for given subpopulations, age groups, and genders. The Alliance has stated:

> There are strong links between the interests of Codex and those of the World Trade Organization (WTO), which can impose heavy fines and sanctions against non-compliant countries. Genuine concern for consumer health and welfare comes second to serving the interests of multinational food and drug companies. Codex poses a direct threat to our freedom to access natural foods, herbs and dietary supplements and to take personal responsibility for our own health and welfare.

Citizens for Health (CFH). According to this non-profit health advocacy group, "Codex intends to protect consumers from 'dangers of nutrients' by effectively restricting access to dietary supplement products. The unintended consequences of this approach undermine individual and social health . . . and limit world trade and product innovation." The organization has also stated:

> The devastation of the world's food supply during World War II was the major impetus for the U.S. to introduce the recommended dietary allowances (RDAs) in 1941. But the RDAs were and are recommended levels consumers can use to gauge the nutritional value or potential health-optimizing benefits of specific products—not mandated or legis-

lated levels established to block U.S. products or consumer access to the health-optimizing levels of innovative, high-potency food supplements. Codex would do well to remember that its core mission is food purity. FAO's mandate, hence Codex's mandate, was not to "dumb down" the potency of nutritional supplements throughout the world. The overriding standards should be these: purity and truthfulness in labeling. Products should state what they contain, contain what they state, the natural or synthetic sources from where they are derived and whether these sources are believed to be genetically engineered (GE or GMO) sources or not. Consumers have the right, and therefore the responsibility, for what they purchase. National governments and Codex should re-focus their efforts on truthful labeling and product purity.

National Health Federation (NHF). This Codex-recognized NGO, which is represented at Codex meetings, has said, "Codex guidelines and standards will inevitably supersede domestic laws, including the Dietary Supplement Health and Education Act of 1994." They have also commented:

[The NHF] opposes the . . . Codex member states who wrongly believe that consumer health will be enhanced by: (1) denying that dietary supplements can benefit normal, healthy people; (2) incorrectly defining dietary supplements as only those vitamins and minerals that the body cannot manufacture itself; (3) restricting the upper-limit amounts of vitamins and minerals, particularly by referring to currently crude and archaic medical beliefs about nutrients; (4) restricting any physiological benefit information for consumers; (5) restricting the lower limit amounts of vitamins and minerals that may be consumed by individuals; and (6) creating "positive" and "negative" lists of dietary supplements . . . [The NHF] supports a supports a Codex process that will free up health knowledge and products for the entire world. A free-market system of choice and knowledge will avoid the errors of central planning that sets standards, however well intentioned, into stone. With the doubling time of knowledge constantly accelerating, mankind cannot afford the 'luxury' of getting stuck in health standards established in the 20th Century while new health knowledge and products are discovered almost daily. The best way to ensure such progress and advancing health is to keep the planners and bureaucrats from straitjacketing dietary supplements with medievalist thinking and restrictions.

Guidelines categorize vitamin and mineral supplements as foods, not drugs. Also, unlike RDAs, the Guidelines do not limit vitamins and minerals contained in supplements to very low amounts. The IADSA expected that the Guidelines would expand global markets for supplement manufacturers.

Yet, not everyone was enthusiastic. Many consumers and manufacturers of dietary supplements feared that the Codex Guidelines would remove important supplement products from the market. According to Jim Turner, "Codex could have adopted the more open provisions of DSHEA as its international guidelines for supplements but did not; instead, it adopted a significantly more restrictive set of principles."

The restrictive nature of the Codex Guidelines is due in part to the influence of the European Union's Food Supplement Directive, which was originally proposed in 2000 and announced in 2002, around the same time as the Codex controversy. The Directive, which was ultimately finalized in 2010, reflects the rigid restrictions of the 1996 German proposal. The fact that some officials simultaneously occupied key positions in the German government, the European Union, and the Codex bureaucracy further inflamed the situation and upset consumer groups. Opponents of the Codex Guidelines noted similarities between the EU's Food Supplements Directive, the Codex Alimentarius Guidelines for Vitamin and Mineral Supplements, and the original German proposal, which created greater worry about future access to supplements.

To encourage other nations to accept their Directive's provisions for supplement regulations, EU leaders touted the Codex Guidelines as a precedent in determining food supplement regulations, a strategy that has also been used by lobbyists in the United States (see the inset on page 112). Supported by the EU, Codex asked its members to formally adopt the EU Food Supplements Directive as national legislation. The only takers thus far have been Belgium and Italy; Belgium has adopted an EU-established list of permitted herbs with specific conditions of use, and in July 2012, Italy adopted a similar list of botanicals that are approved for use in food supplements, along with conditions of use and labeling requirements. This has generated a great deal of confusion for regulators, manufacturers, and consumers.

Facing opposition from both manufacturers and consumers worldwide, the Codex Guidelines issued in 2005 seemed to be as far as the EU could go in terms of extending their supplement-restrictive laws to

The Role of Special Interests

One problem with the Codex system is its relationship with multinational corporate interests. Special interest groups and companies can influence the Codex Commission through non-governmental organizations (NGOs) or national delegations that cater to these multibillion-dollar stakeholders. This relationship is particularly detrimental when it comes to food purity standards.

In addition, there are some important differences between European and U.S. industry groups. First, pharmaceutical and chemical corporations based in European countries, such as Germany and France, produce most of the vitamins, minerals, and botanicals sold across the continent. Therefore, these companies favor low-quality commodity ingredients, like chromium chloride, and questionable additives, such as cyclamates. Second, European trade and consumer groups are much more conciliatory and accommodating than U.S. groups. And finally, European law does not support free speech as strongly as U.S. law. For example, in France, there are restrictions regarding "offending the dignity of the public," which can encompass offenses such as insulting any kind of public servant. In Germany, disparaging the president or government and "casting false suspicion" are considered crimes. Who's to say what actions could fall into these categories?

One telling example of these differences was when, in 2007, the Codex officially adopted nine additives as part of the General Standard for Food Additives (GSFA) at levels proposed by the IADSA. The additives that were approved for use in food supplement products, most of which are synthetic, included acesulfame potassium (K), aspartame, castor oil, cyclamates, neotame, polysorbates, polyvinyl alcohol, saccharin, and sucralose. Previously, in 2006, industry had managed to prevent the deletion of four questionable additives from the Codex General Standard, including erythrosine, a synthetic coal tar dye banned for most uses in Norway and the United States. Industry also reportedly played a role in raising the approved levels of the harmful additives BHA, BHT, and carnauba wax.

Most of the additives that industry groups have advocated over the years are associated with negative, even toxic, side effects, and some additives are even banned in certain countries. Cyclamates, for example, were banned as carcinogenic by the FDA, as well as Britain, Sweden, Denmark, Germany, and Finland in 1969. Acesulfame K stimulates insulin secretion, which may aggravate reactive hypoglycemia. In several studies on rodents, the chemical produced lung and breast tumors, as well as leukemia and chronic respiratory disease, when administered in moderate doses. The Material Safety Data Sheet (MSDS) for acesulfame K indicates that it may be toxic to the kidneys and liver. In addition, there have been concerns that neotame, like aspartame, can gradually lead to neurotoxic and immunotoxic damage because it contains a combination of a formaldehyde metabolite—which is toxic at even extremely low doses—and an excitotoxic amino acid.

According to the Environmental Defense Fund's Chemical Scorecard, polyvinyl alcohol is also suspected to be toxic, particularly to the liver and gastrointestinal and neurological systems. It is most commonly used as a fiber reinforcement in concrete, and as an adhesive or thickener in latex paints, hairsprays, and glues. Although the hazard warning regarding cancer was lifted for saccharin in 2001, questions about the safety of sucralose—a highly processed chemical sweetener—are multiplying. In fact, in 2006, a Citizen Petition called upon the FDA to revoke their approval of sucralose due to its reported adverse effects. It's also worth mentioning that sucralose is produced via a process that releases toxins like cyclohexane into the environment.

Of course, for every report that raises safety concerns about a certain additive, manufacturers produce volumes of supportive data in contradiction. But rather than scrutinize every single artificial compound, we should ask some basic questions: Are U.S. natural products companies truly in support of using synthetic chemical additives? Do international trade organizations properly represent the will of the U.S. dietary supplement industry, or are they more influenced by European "pharma-tritional" interests in their support for certain chemical additives?

the global arena. Today, however, the EU is using other directives, such as the Directive on Traditional Herbal Medicinal Products, to gain more supplement restrictions than the Codex Guidelines provided. Some of their directives contain provisions that seem to interfere with international trade rules, which directly conflicts with the reason for Codex's existence in the first place.

Within this context, many dietary supplement advocates in the United States feel that only DSHEA stands between consumers and international regulations that "dumb down" or take away innovative, high-potency supplements. U.S. supplement companies that sell overseas, suffering from the effects of Codex guidelines and EU directives,

Misinformation Miasma

Few global goings-on have generated as much fear, panic, misinformation, and information that is just plain false as has Codex Alimentarius, especially in the years and months leading up to the 2005 meeting in Rome. Below are some common myths surrounding the Codex, and more importantly, the facts:

MYTH: Your right to sell or buy supplements ended in the summer of 2005.

FACT: In July 2005, Codex adopted vitamin and mineral guidelines that were previously ratified in Germany, in November 2004. As of August 1, 2005, the EU's Food Supplements Directive began restricting (in or into Europe) the sale of dietary supplements containing any ingredient or form of an ingredient that was not on the "approved" lists. The ingredients that received "derogation" status were temporarily excluded from this rule, meaning that they were approved for continued sale in European countries for a limited length of time, and were being considered as potential additions to the list of approved ingredients. Still, despite this temporary grace period for some supplements, European retailers and consumers alike have definitely had their supplement choices curtailed as of August 1, 2005.

MYTH: Dosage limits that will be set are going to be based on an acknowledgment that dietary supplements are inherently benign.

FACT: The dosage levels that Codex will set are going to be largely based on the findings of the FAO/WHO Nutrient Risk Assessment Project. The project is based on a framework typically used for toxic chemicals and environmental hazards, which is obviously not the best model for developing recommended upper-level dosage amounts for dietary supplements.

MYTH: The Directives on supplements and herbs will have no impact on U.S. products.

FACT: When considering this issue, one important but overlooked fact is that some American companies that export products to Europe do not want to have two separate "catalogs" of products. This often leads to the decision to either no longer sell to Europe or, for economic reasons, "dumb down" its supplements to accommodate both markets. This is not a theoretical scenario; according to a few dietary supplement companies with whom I have been in discussion, it is already happening. In addition, according to the FDA, "Other countries with more restrictive laws and regulations for dietary supplement products than the U.S. may create trade barriers to the importation of products manufactured by the U.S. dietary supplement industry."

MYTH: Codex is part of some huge conspiracy to take away our health freedom and our supplements.

FACT: Codex was originally formed with the best of intentions. Nevertheless, what consumer protection means to European regulators is, in many ways, quite different from what that means to the FDA. In Europe, regulators have tradition-ally over-regulated dietary supplements, in many cases classifying supplements as drugs because of what some regard as a coddling, paternalistic "nanny state" approach to consumer protection. Furthermore, there are many international treaties that recognize Codex as the authority on food safety and dietary sup-plements, a complex web of trade-related connections and international recog-nition that will, at least theoretically, give "teeth" to Codex's guidelines.

MYTH: The FDA would never modify its regulations (through rulemaking) to adjust U.S. law to international standards.

FACT: This is not necessarily the case. On October 11, 1995, the FDA stated that they intended to "increase its efforts to harmonize its regulatory require-ments with those of foreign governments." The FDA also noted, "If the agency concludes that it is appropriate to propose to revise its regulations to accom-modate consideration of Codex standards, FDA plans to . . . outline specific revisions." Although attorney Justin J. Prochnow has observed that these state-ments are "not akin to mandated FDA policy," ten years later, the FDA still seemed to be moving towards harmonization, as suggested by an agency statement in 2005: "Failure to reach a consistent, harmonized set of laws, reg-ulations and standards within the free trade agreements and the World Trade Organization Agreements can result in considerable economic repercussions."

MYTH: Codex will never get involved in the World Trade Organization's international trade disputes.

FACT: The WTO has stated that Codex "can be called in as experts to give advice to WTO dispute settlement panels."

MYTH: Codex, like other international guidelines, does not have regulations and is only voluntary.

FACT: Although this is true in theory, the reality has been aptly summed up by the WTO:

Before the entry into force of the WTO, international standards, guidelines, recommendations and other advisory texts could be adopted by governments on a voluntary basis. Although these norms remain voluntary, a new status has been conferred on them by the SPS [Agreement on the Application of Sanitary and Phytosanitary Measures]. A WTO Member adopting such norms is presumed to be in full compliance with the SPS Agreement.

Lending further proof, Prochnow has pointed to Article 3 of the SPS agreement, which reads, "To harmonize sanitary and phytosanitary measures on as wide a basis as possible, Members *shall* base their [food safety] measures on international standards, guidelines or recommendations" (emphasis mine). Prochnow notes that the use of the word *shall* "effectively makes the 'voluntary' Codex guidelines mandatory for Member Nations of the WTO," including the United States.

MYTH: If the WTO was to impose sanctions on the United States, the U.S. would have to automatically change its laws to comply.

FACT: This is technically false. If the WTO imposed sanctions against the U.S. for a specific case of non-adherence to Codex guidelines in international trade, the U.S., according to Prochnow, would have to decide whether or not the sanctions were burdensome enough to call for harmonization with Codex guidelines. However, in order for the law to be changed, Congress would have to use the standard legislative process.

MYTH: The FDA can quickly and easily adopt Codex guidelines as new regulations.

FACT: If the FDA wanted to implement "Codex-friendly" supplement regulations that would not undermine DSHEA, the agency would have to follow standard agency protocol. The first step would be to issue a Notice of Proposed Rule-making (NOPR), which would likely generate a massive consumer response depending on the nature of the proposal.

MYTH: Nothing good came out of the July 2005 Rome meeting.

FACT: A positive result of the Rome meeting in 2005, and a piece of news that received hardly any press, was the WHO Global Strategy on Diet, Physical Activity and Health. This strategy, which was endorsed by the World Health Assembly, was developed at the request of WHO member countries to reduce

> disease and death linked to nutritional and lifestyle factors. The Global Strategy calls for Codex to "continue to give full consideration . . . to evidence-based action it might take to improve the health standards of foods." In a discussion paper (Document CAC 28/ LIM/6), the WHO said that this Global Strategy "reflects an international public health initiative" intended to improve world health and reduce obesity, heart disease, cancer, and diabetes, which are—as the WHO acknowledged—partly "determined by nutrition and dietary choices." The WHO's Global Strategy initiative represents a critical recommitment to health on behalf of Codex's parent organizations. It is also an unparalleled opportunity for the health freedom movement to become constructively and meaningfully involved in the development of the Global Strategy at the Codex committee level.

now feel compelled to dumb down their formulas or reduce their potencies in order to accommodate both the U.S. and European markets; the cost of creating completely different formulas for domestic and international sales is too daunting and expensive for most companies. Moreover, because most companies lack the additional resources needed to legally challenge EU regulations and Codex guidelines, they have been marginalized in the global debate.

Still, many pro-supplement advocates and natural product industry associations have been able persuade Congress to prohibit the FDA from harmonizing its supplement rules with Codex. The provisions of DSHEA can be changed only through formal legal action on the part of the U.S. government, which has neither been proposed nor attempted. As long as DSHEA and anti-harmonization legislation remains in place, Codex guidelines will not be adopted by the United States.

The controversy surrounding supplement regulation brings to light the debate between biochemical individuality—the idea that each person has unique needs when it comes to nutritional intake—versus the notion of dietary standards that can be applied to most individuals, as reflected by Codex, the EU, and U.S. RDAs. Whereas the principle of biochemical individuality allows for a highly diversified supplement market, imposing dietary standards results in a market with fewer product options, but, as some marketers believe, more customers and sales. These cookie-cutter standards are vehemently opposed by members of the health freedom community who unanimously support the importance of biochemical individuality and the rights of individuals to pursue what they consider to be optimal nutrient intake for themselves. This struggle for health freedom continues even today.

CONCLUSION

The debate over the regulation of dietary supplements will doubtless continue in various forums. Unfortunately, Codex is a forum in which policy debates are dominated by powerful economic interests and governments. Groups representing consumers and small businesses are essentially blocked from having a serious influence on these debates. Nevertheless, the excluded groups have demonstrated an ability to influence international food policy through community organizing at the grassroots level. It is here at the local level that concerned citizens who lack the power and money of large institutions can make a significant difference.

There are a few important principles that should guide this effort. The overriding standards for food and food supplements should be purity and truthfulness in labeling. Products should state what they contain and contain what they claim. They should list the natural or synthetic sources from which they are derived, and whether these sources are believed to be genetically engineered. National governments and CODEX should focus, or re-focus, its efforts on product purity and transparency.

Consumers can get a safer, healthier, and more reasonably priced food supply if they demand it. An industry veteran put it this way: "The industry has done a great job moving the ball to the forty-yard line and has gone as far as it possibly can." It is now up to consumers to carry the ball to the goal line, and it is up to consumer groups to help them do so.

5

The Canada Example

*"Canadians can be radical, but they must be radical in their
own peculiar way, and that way must be in harmony
with our national traditions and ideals."*

—AGNES MACPHAIL, SPEECH AT THE CANADIAN CLUB,
TORONTO, ONTARIO (MARCH 4, 1935)

So far, this book has discussed the natural health movement in the
United States both on its own and within the context of global-
ism. Now it's important to take a look at what is happening to
Canada, our northern neighbor, in order to gain a firmer understanding of what is at stake in the fight for health freedom. Although aboriginal healing traditions are engrained in the history of both Canada
and the U.S., Canadians have generally been more forward-thinking in
terms of herbal medicine and natural healing. At the same time, however, the Canadian government has been much more restrictive than
the United States when it comes to dietary supplements and other natural health products. This fact is likely due to Canada's comparative-
ly strong cultural, social, and political ties to Europe, which has also
been more progressive in terms of naturopathic medicine and yet more
prohibitive towards supplements. Today, the country is at a crossroads;
it must choose more restrictions or more freedom of choice. This chapter explores Canada's natural health history and current policies as an
example—and a warning—to the United States as it wages its own battles with the FDA.

CANADA'S NATURAL HEALTH HISTORY

Natural medicine has a defined place in Canada's history and culture, as it was practiced and developed by the country's aboriginal peoples over thousands of years. It was through these societies that European settlers in Canada first encountered traditional medicine and healing practices.

One of the most famous examples is that of the French explorer Jacques Cartier, whose ships became ice-bound in their moorings during his Second Voyage in 1536. The combination of drifting snows, bitter cold, and inadequate nutrition led to an outbreak of scurvy among Cartier's 110-man crew. By the time Cartier encountered the native people that ultimately saved them, eight men had already died, fifty men were close to death, and the others—with the exception of three or four individuals—were sick. According to Stephen Leacock in 1915:

It happened one day that Cartier was walking up and down by himself upon the ice when he saw a band of Indians coming over to him from Stadacona [near present-day Quebec City]. Among them was the interpreter, Dom Agaya, whom Cartier had known to be stricken with the illness only ten days before, but who now appeared to be in abundant health. On being asked the manner of his cure, the interpreter told Cartier that he had been healed by a beverage made from the leaves and bark of a tree.

This "beverage" was a tea made from juniper bark and pine needles. According to historian Toni Leland, a few members of Cartier's crew accepted the tea, finding themselves relieved of their symptoms almost instantly. When they realized the tea's curative abilities, wrote Leland, the rest of the men were "ready to kill one another" in order to obtain the "miracle potion."

Leacock noted that Cartier afterwards wrote, "If all the doctors of Lorraine and Montpellier had been there with all the drugs of Alexandria, they could not have done as much in a year as the said tree did in six days." It would be another 200 years before the actual cause of scurvy, as well its connection to vitamin C, would be discovered by James Lind, a Scottish Naval surgeon.

Another famous example of natural medicine in Canadian history revolves around Rene Caisse, a well-respected surgical nurse in

Haileybury, Ontario in the first part of the twentieth century. According to author Gary L. Glum, in 1922, an elderly female patient told Caisse that she had been cured of what was presumed to be cancer with a traditional herbal remedy. According to her story, years earlier, the woman had experienced pain and swelling in her breast, and was told by an Ojibwa medicine man that it was cancer. She first sought treatment from conventional doctors, who recommended surgery to remove the breast tumors—a risky, expensive procedure. Instead, she accepted treatment from the medicine man, who gave her a tea consisting of blessed thistle, burdock root, kelp, red clover, sheep sorrel, slippery elm bark, Turkey rhubarb root, and water cress. According to Glum, the woman told Caisse that she drank the tea every day, and gradually her tumors were reduced in size until they disappeared altogether. She had been cancer-free ever since.

Caisse, fascinated by the woman's apparent cure, wrote down the herbs used in the tea. "I knew that doctors threw up their hands when cancer was discovered in a patient; it was the same as a death sentence, just about," she recounted some years later. "I decided that if I should ever develop cancer, I would use this herb tea."

Months later, Caisse received word that her aunt had undergone surgery to treat stomach cancer. Unfortunately, the surgery was unsuccessful, as the disease had advanced and spread to her liver. Her aunt's doctor, R. O. Fisher, informed her that she would live another six months at most. Caisse asked the doctor's permission to give her aunt the herbal remedy under his supervision, and he agreed. Caisse's aunt took the tea for about two months, and gradually regained her strength. Eventually, she made a full recovery and lived another twenty-one years. Caisse later wrote, "Dr. Fisher was so impressed that he asked me to use my treatment on some of his other hopeless patients." Over the next decade, it became known that Caisse and Dr. Fisher were, in fact, treating cancer patients with the tea and that they "showed enough improvement to convince Dr. Fisher that Rene Caisse was on to an important discovery," wrote Glum. Fisher thus became one of her strongest supporters. In fact, according to Caisse, it was Fisher who first suggested that they administer the tea hypodermically (via the skin) to achieve better results.

In 1926, nine licensed Canadian physicians, amazed by Caisse's success, petitioned the Department of Health and Welfare to allow

Suppression of Traditional Medicine

Today, it is well known that many traditional Native American remedies are actually similar to—or form the basis of—many common pharmaceutical products. Nevertheless, in Canada, traditional medicine has not been universally accepted. Even though European herbal traditions were brought to Canada by early explorers and settlers, there was a good degree of skepticism among the general population when it came to indigenous healing practices. With the exception of early explorers like Jacques Cartier, many of the first European settlers in Canada frowned upon native healing practices, believing their medical knowledge to be superior. The results of this attitude were summed up by Dr. Raymond Obomsawin in his book *Traditional Medicine for Canada's First Peoples* (2007):

> Similar to many indigenous nations of the world, the Aboriginal people of Canada . . . [were progressively] coerced into abandoning their traditional ideologies and practices in relation to health care. As the European settlers became the predominant population of Canada, their health care systems assumed the right to declare what was "acceptable" practice for all of society. Blatant disregard, and perhaps true ignorance, for the consequences that this major shift in health ideologies would impose on the Aboriginal population of Canada resulted in an almost complete loss of Aboriginal traditional medicine.

The shift to conventional, or mainstream, medicine led to the dismissal or marginalization of many traditional healing methods, which was regarded as unscientific quackery. This new hierarchy of medicine forced native peoples to give up their own ways and adopt what accepted practices of mainstream medicine. As generations of knowledge went unused, indigenous peoples not only lost an important part of their identity, but were also made vulnerable to illnesses and other conditions that could have been effectively treated with traditional methods.

This suppression continues today. Although Canada strives to have one of the best healthcare systems in the world, native people have inadequate access to medical care, especially services for mental health and substance abuse. This is a serious problem, as suicide rates are five to six times higher among indigenous populations than the general population, according to Grand Chief Doug Kelly, chair of the First Nations Health Council.

Moreover, anyone who has ever sought traditional treatment in Canada knows that it is not government-funded, which forces people to get care from only conventional practitioners that are covered (and supported) by the health-care system. According to the 2011 official Traditional Healers Gathering Report:

Traditional medicine as well as naturopathic medicine and other forms of alternative medicines are not currently funded through the Provincial or Federal government of Canada. There are some instances where portions of a visit to a practitioner or alternative medicine and laboratory testing will be covered but, as a whole, naturopathic physicians do not bill the government or government funded health organizations. This makes it very challenging for patients to utilize the health care that they prefer. It also makes it very challenging for organizations or clinics to hire traditional healers or naturopathic physicians.

Yet, despite the growth of conventional and organized medicine, as well as the ongoing suppression of traditional healing, the public has once again discovered holistic and alternative methods. Renewed interest in traditional remedies and treatments has resulted in efforts to revive native healing techniques and include other alternative forms, such as Traditional Chinese Medicine (TCM) and Ayurveda, in the healthcare system. Unfortunately, the government continues to pass legislation that restricts the treatments and products available to the Canadian population. These regulations affect not only traditional herbal medicine, but also any product considered to be a natural health product, or NHP.

large-scale tests of the herbal remedy, which she called "Essiac"—Caisse spelled backwards. While the petition demonstrated support for Essiac and the promise of natural medicine in general, it also marked the beginning of an institutional war on Essiac tea, waged primarily by the government and mainstream medical establishment. As Caisse wrote in the *Bracebridge Examiner:*

This was the beginning of nearly 50 years of persecution by those in authority, from the government to the medical profession, that I endured in trying to help those afflicted with cancer. However, when these two doctors sent from Ottawa found that I was working with nine of the most eminent physicians in Toronto, and was giving my treatment only at their request, and under their observation, they did not arrest me. . . . I later moved to Peterborough, east of Toronto, and lived in a rented house, where I was no sooner moved in than the College of Physicians and Surgeons sent a health officer to issue a warrant for my arrest, again the charge was "practising medicine without a licence." I have lost count of the number of times I have been threatened with arrest and imprisonment for treating patients with Essiac. . . . I never dreamed of the opposition and the persecution that would be my lot in trying to help suffering humanity with no thought of personal gain. I have never claimed that my treatment cures cancer—although many of my patients and the doctors with whom I have worked claim that it does.

Despite this persecution, Caisse worked with the well-known Brusch Clinic in the 1960s. According to Campaign for Truth in Medicine, Dr. Charles A. Brusch, the personal physician for President John F. Kennedy, cured his own bowel cancer using only Essiac tea. He researched the herbal tea for a decade and came to the conclusion that "Essiac is a cure for cancer, period. All studies done at laboratories in the United States and Canada support this conclusion."

Encounters with traditional healing knowledge, such as that of Caisse and Cartier, resulted in groundbreaking discoveries in herbal medicine. Their stories demonstrate the receptiveness of many Canadians to these practices in spite of efforts to suppress them. Caisse's Ojibwa recipe was met with disdain by the medical establishment not because it was reported to be curative, but rather because it was a botanical remedy, not a pharmaceutical. This pro-pharmaceutical attitude shaped the healthcare system in Canada and influenced government regulations of natural health products.

THE DEVELOPMENT OF ORGANIZED MEDICINE AND HEALTHCARE

Until the nineteenth century, Canadians were generally left to their own devices when it came to medical treatment, as there was no real need for a nationwide healthcare system. Typically, family members or self-taught village healers were responsible for caring for those who required medical attention. Common treatment methods were usually passed down from one generation to the next, either by word-of-mouth or written journals, and they did not change much until the 1800s. When change did come, though, it came fast and furious. In a short period of time, the ways in which people were treated in Canada changed dramatically.

There were a few different reasons for the sudden change. First, beginning in the early 1800s, there was an influx of immigrants to Canada, mostly from the United States and Great Britain, which gave way to significant population growth. Second, in the 1820s, there was an increase in the number of medical schools in Canada, particularly in the country's northern region. The first medical school was founded in 1824 in Montreal, which today is known as the Faculty of Medicine of McGill University.

Advances in medicine also contributed to the changes in healthcare. As people became more aware of the differences between charlatans and professionals with actual medical knowledge, more efforts were made to regulate the field. Debate ensued over how the medical profession should be defined, and whether or not medical degrees and licenses should be required in order to practice. During the 1860s, conventional doctors practicing *allopathy*—the modern system of medicine whereby disease is combated with the use of remedies like drugs and surgery—tried to assert their authority by advocating new registration and licensing methods for doctors. This made it increasingly difficult for homeopaths and Eclectic physicians to qualify for practice. The medical profession was more or less formally defined when the Canadian Medical Association was born in 1867. Two years later, the Ontario Medical Act gave power to the College of Physicians and Surgeons of Ontario to review and test its graduates to qualify them for medical practice.

Epidemics also played a major role in the development of organized medicine and healthcare in Canada during the 1800s. Cholera especially presented a problem to the U.S. and Canadian populations, which were affected by outbreaks in 1832, 1834, 1849, and throughout the 1850s. Although European researchers, such as Filippo Pacini and Robert Koch, proved that cholera was linked to germs and hygiene, physicians continued to treat the disease using harsh and ineffective methods like cauterizing, bleeding, and excessive amounts of drugs like opium.

In response to the cholera epidemic and the unsatisfactory ways in which it was treated, the first localized boards of health were established. The purpose of these boards was to enforce new sanitation laws that were meant to stop future outbreaks of contagious diseases due to unsanitary conditions and poor hygiene. At the same time, treatment centers similar to modern-day hospitals were springing up all over the country.

Despite this progress, it was clear that the well-being of patients was not always the first priority. Therefore, many Canadians remained largely dissatisfied and still open to new ideas, such as naturopathy, as they were introduced by European immigrants.

THE DECLINE OF NATUROPATHY AND RISE OF MAINSTREAM MEDICINE

Naturopathy became one of the most important healing systems in Canada during the 1800s and paved the way for complementary modalities like homeopathy, osteopathy, and chiropractic methods. As noted in Chapter One, the man credited with starting this movement is Benedict Lust, a German immigrant who advocated natural healing techniques in the U.S. from the late 1800s through the early 1900s. His philosophy piqued the interest of many Canadians, who welcomed Lust's ideas and began to seek natural remedies for diseases to avoid harsh treatments that were commonly practiced.

In many ways, the Canadian and American interest in natural healing mirrored each other and developed in a similar pattern. According to Dr. Iva Lloyd, author of *The History of Naturopathic Medicine: A Canadian Perspective* (2009), between 1896 and the 1920s, at the same time that naturopathy was flourishing in the United States, "naturopathic medicine steadily developed: the number of colleges increased; regulation was achieved in four provinces." In other words, naturopathic physicians were able to obtain licenses and fulfill other requirements necessary for practicing medicine.

Unfortunately, thanks to the efforts of pro-pharmaceutical advocates, the Canadian government soon imposed restrictions on natural medicine. When these forces banded together, it was difficult for naturopathic physicians to adequately fight the skeptical view of natural medicine that was becoming engrained in the rapidly evolving allopathic healthcare system. Eventually, naturopathic doctors lost the privileges they had once shared with conventional physicians. For example, Sir Victor Sassoon, a British philanthropist who reportedly "had regained his health as a result of naturopathic treatments," was rejected when he offered to finance a "Chair of Naturopathic Medicine" at the University of British Columbia in 1943. According to Lloyd, "His check was returned and his offer refused."

Naturopathic medicine declined as quickly as it had appeared, though other health-related movements continued in both the U.S. and Canada, including the right-living movement, the clean-eating movement, and the temperance movement. By the mid-1950s, naturopathic education in Canada was almost extinct due to "lack of funding, opposition and struggles with other systems of medicine." Although steps were taken to replace toxic patent remedies with safer, regulated pharmaceuticals, naturopathic medicine was legally and economically suppressed in Canada for several decades. Naturopathy didn't regain popularity in Canada again until the 1970s, which was due in part to the so-called Hippie Movement's emphasis on nutrition and the environment, as well as a "reawakening to the value of personal responsibility."

In 1989, a meeting in Ontario brought about a unified definition of naturopathic medicine and descriptions of naturopathy's key principles, which were later accepted by the Canadian Naturopathic Association and the American Association of Naturopathic Practitioners.

THE NATURAL HEALTH INDUSTRY
AND THE RISE OF THE HEALTH CANADA AGENCY

Despite the rise of allopathic medicine and the simultaneous suppression of naturopathy, a large portion of the Canadian population continued to be interested in health. Thus, people quickly recognized the link between wellness and nutrition, a realization that marked the beginning of the natural foods movement in Canada. As explained in Chapter One, the movement gained momentum in North America during the early 1900s and eventually came to support not only natural foods, but also all types of natural health products (NHPs), including vitamins, minerals, natural remedies, and other health-promoting substances from plants with medicinal qualities.

Today, there is a wide variety of natural health products. As John R. Harrison stated in his 2008 book, *International Regulation of Natural Health Products*:

> Natural health products (NHPs) are big business both in Canada and elsewhere in the world. The majority of Canadian products previously registered as non-prescription medicines are now NHPs. Consumers are buying these products in record volumes all in an effort to make themselves feel better, get better, and possibly live longer. The NHP industry shows no signs of fading. [Surveys] reveal that more than 50 percent of Canadians are consuming NHPs.

More current statistics show that this percentage has increased. A recent study carried out by the global research company Ipsos-Reid showed that 71 percent of Canadians have used a natural health product, and that 77 percent agree that NHPs can be used to maintain or help achieve good health. And yet most NHPs are unavailable in Canada today, which is due in large part to restrictions imposed by Health Canada, the agency created to oversee issues related to public health, including the regulation of foods, drugs, and natural health products. Established in 1996, Health Canada's stated mission is to protect the national public health, which is why their authority has been extended to natural health products. But because supplements can have effects on the body and, moreover, are made by companies looking to make a profit, the government deemed it necessary to create rules and regulations for NHPs in order to protect the well-being of Canadians. Unfortunately, there were few rules and regulations to protect the Canadian people from the government and other regulatory authorities. As a result, Health Canada has been successful in its efforts to implement laws that go against the wishes of the majority of Canadians.

The timeline below explains how regulations have affected the sale and consumption of natural health products in Canada, from 1920 to the present. Learning about these major milestones in chronological order makes it is easier to notice the pattern these regulations have followed, understand how they have spiraled out of control, and recognize the problems currently facing Canadians who support and prefer natural health alternatives.

The Food and Drugs Act

Canada's relatively short political, legislative, and regulatory history for supplements and natural health products began with the passage of the Food and Drugs Act in 1920, an act that remains the most comprehensive health-related legislation ever passed in Canada. The precursor to this act was the Inland Revenue Act of 1875, which was the first nationwide legislation targeting drugs, food, and alcohol.

Whereas previous laws were modeled on similar acts passed in Great Britain, the Food and Drugs Act was more akin to the U.S. Food and Drugs Act of 1906. In addition to encompassing more products and implementing more regulations, the act—which was formally entitled "An Act respecting food, drugs, cosmetics and therapeutic devices"—also gave the government more power to control every aspect of food, health, and cosmetic products and devices, including their import, export, labeling, advertising, sale, and approval. The act also allowed for quality testing and grading of products, as well as imposing punishments on companies that used false or misleading labeling.

Countless items, including natural health products, still fall under the scope of the Food and Drugs Act, which was updated in 1953. This version of the act placed health products into four categories: drugs, devices, cosmetics, and foods. In fact, an entire section of the act is dedicated to natural health product regulations (NHPRs), which provide guidelines for NHP labeling and require manufacturers to obtain a license before selling any product classified as an NHP. By treating NHPs like a subset of drugs, Health Canada has been able to remove a majority of NHPs from store shelves.

1990—Closure of a World-Class Food Safety and NHP Lab

In 1990, Health Canada shut down one of the world's most renowned food safety labs. The lab, which was headed by one of the most respected natural health experts, Dr. Dennis Awang, was responsible for testing various foods, supplements, and NHPs to determine if they were safe for human consumption. Health Canada decided that the costs associated with running the lab were not justifiable, however, as the vast majority of NHPs did not pose a health risk to the public.

1995—Pharmaceutical Regulations and Natural Health Products

As previously explained, prior to this year, natural health products did not have their own set of regulations and were thus treated as pharmaceutical drugs. Complaints against NHPs were rarely registered, however, so the natural health industry was generally left alone. But this all changed in 1995 when Health Canada suddenly focused its attention on the tens of thousands of NHPs available in Canada. The majority of these products became illegal, which meant that many Canadians could no longer use the NHPs that they once had. The actions taken by Health Canada were legally permissible under the pretext that NHPs were not in compliance with licensing and registration regulations that were already in place for pharmaceuticals. Still, this explanation was insufficient, as NHPs were considered to be extremely safe. According to the Natural Health Products Protection Association (NHPPA):

> Although unregulated, NHPs were not posing a safety risk. Several federal laws prevented fraud or adulteration. In all of Canadian history there has not been a single death caused by a NHP. To understand how significant this is, we only have to compare the NHP track record with some over-the-counter pain medications or common foods such as nuts and shellfish. These common medications/foods kill a number of Canadians each year, including children. More are hospitalized. At the same time, although they carry a risk, we do not ban or over-regulate common medications/foods because we do not consider the risk high enough.

Most Canadians realized that dietary supplements and natural health products were intrinsically benign, while pharmaceutical drugs and synthetic chemicals were intrinsically dangerous. Therefore, they were not favorably disposed towards a restrictive drug-like system for natural products.

1997—Protests and the Charter of Health Freedom

The people of Canada did not intend to take the actions of Health Canada sitting down. Consumers wanted to be able to make their own choices when it came to issues of health and medical treatment. The petition submitted to Parliament in 1997 clearly conveyed this message to the Canadian government, and the movement that followed is considered to be one of the largest in the country's history. The public demonstrated its support for the natural health industry, as well as a desire to freely choose supplements and other NHPs over pharmaceutical products. A parliamentary aide noted, "More Canadians signed the petition to protect their access to NHPs than any petition in Canadian history."

Their efforts were successful, as Canada's Minister of Health, Alan Rock, ordered Health Canada to reevaluate policies governing natural health products. In addition, legislation known as the Charter of Health Freedom was proposed, which was meant to give natural health products their own set of laws and regulations. The charter would prevent government agencies like Health Canada from using shrewd tactics and legal loopholes to pull NHPs off the market. The best description of this legislation can be found at www.charterof healthfreedom.org, where it is stated:

> The Charter protects our access to Natural Health Products and Traditional Medicines by creating a separate legal category for them. Rather than being deemed as dangerous drugs under the Food and Drugs Act, under the Charter Natural Health Products and Traditional Medicines are deemed to be safe, as they are in the United States.

In sum, the charter would provide an appropriate way of handling situations involving NHPs, making it possible to keep safe NHPs on the market and available to the public. At the same time, the government would be able to legally remove potentially harmful NHPs from the market. This would have been a win-win situation for everyone, but getting the charter passed proved to be easier in theory than in reality.

1997—Consultations with the Public

Due to the growing popularity of NHPs and the public opposition to strict regulations, the Canadian government conducted a review of natural health products in October 1997. The goal of the review, which was done by the House of Commons Standing Committee on Health, was to come up with a solution that would satisfy both the public's desire to use NHPs and Health Canada's concerns for consumer safety.

Between October 1997 and April 1998, the Committee consulted with a variety of parties, including individual NHP advocates, health-care professionals, consumer groups, herbalists, and industry-related organizations. Overall, the review was comprehensive.

1998—The Standing Committee's Report

Taking into account the interests of all consulted parties, in May 1998, the Standing Committee of Health submitted their final report, which was entitled, "Regulatory Framework for Natural Health Products." The report consisted of fifty-three recommendations for a new customized set of regulations for NHPs, which included a new definition of natural health products; a stipulation that NHPs be allowed to use health claims, risk-reduction claims, and treatment claims; and the requirement that indigenous healers be allowed to use traditional remedies without interference.

The Natural Health Products Directorate (NHPD)

Once the Health Minister accepted all fifty-three recommendations, the Natural Health Products Directorate (NHPD) was created to deal with matters concerning natural health products. Specifically, their goal was to protect freedom of choice and ensure that Canadians had access to NHPs. Ultimately, however, the NHPD actually managed to restrict access to natural health products and reduce freedom of choice. The truth about the Natural Health Product Directorate was succinctly described by Marilyn Nelson on behalf of Natural Health Freedom Canada:

> The NHPD is accomplishing the exact opposite of the professed objective. It has restricted thousands of safe and effective products from the market, causing some domestic suppliers to go out of

business and others to cut back on their product lines. A number of U.S. companies have also withdrawn their safe and effective products from the Canadian market because the NPN [Natural Product Number] requirements were too much cost and bother for them. Consumers have less freedom to choose safe and effective HPs [health products] than ever before.

The NHPD, therefore, is similar to the FDA in its efforts to shrink the natural products market by making it more difficult for innovative, high-potency supplements to become licensed and available in Canada.

2000—A Healthcare Bombshell

Two years after the recommendations had been accepted, the NHP industry found out that all fifty-three recommendations had been changed and reworked. This discovery was due to the release of a document called "Standards of Evidence and Good Manufacturing Practice," which announced that the government would be adopting and enforcing a drug-regulatory model for NHPs. When word got out, meetings were organized by the NHPD to get feedback and advice from all stakeholders—including consumers, practitioners, and manufacturers—regarding the recommendations. In total, more than 2,100 stakeholders participated in the meetings.

2002—Continued Efforts by the NHP Industry

In 2002, companies in the NHP industry, backed by the Canadian people, actively pushed to have the fifty-three recommendations of the Standing Committee implemented. Even though these recommendations were made years earlier, they had not yet been enforced. According to the NHPPA, ongoing meetings between prominent industry stakeholders and Health Canada confirmed that the new regulatory framework would not be implemented, as Health Canada believed that its goals could be achieved under the regulatory model for drugs.

2002—Cooperation Between Canada and the European Union

This year marked another milestone for the Canadian health and supplement industry. Unfortunately, it was not a positive milestone, but rather a slew of proposed bills that, if enacted, would give the government the power to adopt the laws of foreign countries and international bodies, such as the European Union. This, in turn, would increase the influence and decision-making power of foreign trade groups and organizations when it came to Canadian policies. More worrisome was the fact that the bills would allow the government to adopt foreign laws without the knowledge, vote, or consent of Canadian citizens. While this may seem like a far-fetched scenario, it is actually a far more realistic possibility than many realize. In fact, as mentioned in Chapter Four, it has already happened in Italy.

To make matters worse, Canada and the European Union started down the path of harmonization, a term given to the process in which a country adjusts its own sovereign laws and regulations to the mirror that of other countries. Specifically, Health Canada intended to harmonize its policies with that of the International Conference on Harmonization of Technical Requirements of Pharmaceuticals for Human Use, or ICH. As Health Canada states on its website, "Health Canada, as official observer to and active participant in the International Conference on Harmonisation (ICH), is committed to the adoption and implementation of ICH guidances and standards." The main danger of harmonization, aside from compromising national sovereignty, is that standards, regulations, and laws almost always become more restrictive rather than reflect a more free-market approach.

2004—New NHP Regulations

Beginning in January 2004, a whole new set of regulations for natural health products became law. In *International Regulation of Natural Health Products* (2008), John R. Harrison summarized the new legal definition of natural health products:

> [The] new regulations define NHPs for regulatory and legislative purposes as vitamins, minerals, herbs, homeopathic products, traditional medicines, probiotics, amino acids, essential fatty acids and extracts or isolates from plant and animal matter. These are the substances that will be legally considered NHPs.

On the one hand, having an exact, explicit definition of an NHP was a good thing, as a vague definition could lead to uncertainty on the part of supplement makers and retailers, as well as a tendency to over-reach on the part of regulators. On the other hand, however, the new framework gave Health Canada the means to continually add products to the NHP list or deliberately not include others, effectively keeping them off the market. In other words, there was a potentially endless list of products that could legally be considered NHPs, and few limitations on power of the NHPD to decide what products could and could not be included on the list.

In mid-2004, in an effort to deflect the harsh new regulations, health advocates sponsored Bill C-420, an act that would have formally recognized NHPs as food supplements, thereby exempting them from drug-like regulations. The bill was ultimately dismissed.

2004 to 2006—The Mass Disappearance of Natural Health Products

Even though the new NHPRs (effective January 1, 2004) were intended to protect the rights of Canadians to buy natural health products, they actually had the opposite effect. Because the NHPRs enforced the drug-regulatory model, natural health products, subjected to many of the same rules, began to mysteriously vanish from store shelves. The NHPD required reviews of pre-market license applications for every product, as well as site-license applications for all supplement manufacturers, packagers, labelers, and companies that imported to Canada. In other words, every product had to be cleared by the NHPD and issued a license before it could be sold in Canada. In addition, any company that manufactured, packaged, or labeled products in Canada had to have a license for their place, or site, of business.

Furthermore, in order to receive product pre-approval, supplement makers had to submit evidence to the NHPD documenting safety, proper manufacturing, and data supporting any health claims. But as the NHPD became flooded with submissions, a backlog of applications was created. As a result, many companies were left in limbo as to whether their products could be sold in Canada.

2007—Ban on American Natural Health Products

Even more natural health products began to disappear in Canada when, in 2007, more than 20,000 NHPs imported from the United

States were officially blocked from entering the Canadian market. Additionally, a provision of the 2004 NHPRs took effect, which banned some American companies from exporting to Canada unless they applied for licenses. However, these companies decided to save their time and money, and stopped exports to Canada altogether. The thousands of products that disappeared from Canadian stores became classified as "Schedule F drugs"—drugs requiring a prescription.

2008—The Unleashing of Bill C-51

Despite the regulations on NHPs, 95 percent of natural health products on store shelves were still unlicensed in 2008. To make it clear that this would no longer be tolerated, Parliament introduced Bill C-51, an amendment to the existing Food and Drugs Act. On the surface, Bill C-51 did not seem to be overly restrictive, but upon closer inspection, it was obvious that the sole purpose of the bill was to remove more NHPs from the market and prevent new ones from entering it. According to Shane Starling in a 2008 article, the true goal of this bill was to "make it more difficult for dietary supplements to achieve natural health product status by subjecting them to costly pharma-style registration procedures."

Not only would the bill have made it more difficult for companies to have NHPs licensed in Canada, it also would have made it illegal for private citizens to share their own NHPs without a license. According to the legal definition of a natural health product, this rule could have been applied to common foods and ingredients, from cranberries to garlic. Moreover, to avoid harsh penalties and lengthy licensing procedures, many companies would have been forced to stop producing new NHPs altogether. In other words, innovation would be completely stifled.

2009—Removal of Multi-Ingredient Health Formulas from the Market

Any hope of seeing a clear path to approval for multi-ingredient health products was crushed in 2009, when it became well known that the industry lacked proper ways for approving NHPs containing more than a single ingredient. According to the NHPPA, Natural Product Numbers (NPNs) had largely been given only to single-ingredient products. "There is no suitable mechanism for the NHPD to evaluate multi-ingredient formulations," noted the NHPPA. "It is these products that form a larger component of NHP products currently on store shelves. The challenge is that to properly evaluate these multi-ingredient products there is an inadequate timeline in place before enforcement action comes into effect."

Since the crackdown on natural health products began, advocates for NHPs and the companies that produce them have been pushing for more favorable regulations that respect the rights of Canadian citizens. As of 2010, seven years after the passage of the NHPRs, there was a massive backlog of NHP product-license applications that had not yet been reviewed by Health Canada. Because new products were technically barred from the marketplace, there has been little innovation since 2004 and few new NHPs. The industry outcry over this logjam led to the Natural Health Products (Unprocessed Product Application) Regulations (NHP UPLAR), which allowed companies to market their products while awaiting pre-approval as long as the products met certain criteria and eventually underwent post-market oversight. In other words, if products were approved before they were introduced and then assessed after they were on store shelves, they would be allowed to remain on the market. Unfortunately, NHP UPLAR expires as of February 2013, which is when it was decided that the NHPD would theoretically be able to eliminate the backlog.

THE FIGHT IS NOT OVER

The controversy over natural health products in Canada continues today. By most accounts, Health Canada has misused its powers and misled the natural health industry, as well as the public, about NHP regulations. According to the advocacy group Natural Health Freedom Canada (NHFC), "There is a long list of items used by Health Canada (going back to 1994) to trick the public into thinking changes that weaken health protection laws and regulations are somehow going to strengthen safety." The most recent example of this is Health Canada's "Technical Discussions on Regulatory Modernization," which took place in 2010 and 2011 and consisted of three different events, all of which involved some form of deception. For instance, they used vague terminology like "transition" and "risk management" to sugarcoat changes that would ultimately be detrimental to the public well-being. As written on the NHFC website, "Transition was a word used to describe an attempt to get rid of safety rights in the Food and Drugs Act. The attempt failed after we decoded transition as meaning abdication of legal duty."

Nevertheless, today there is a long list of supplements and health products that are classified as drugs and, therefore, no longer available to the public. Many of these products—a list that includes DHEA, kava kava, L-carnitine, L-tryptophan, and natural progesterone—were available for many years in Canada and continue to be available in other countries without incident.

Health Canada's stated reasons for banning these products are somewhat suspicious. According to an article posted on NHPPA'S Charter of Health Freedom website:

> Within the last four years, more than 40,000 NHPs have been removed from the market. These NHPs include vitamins, minerals, EFAs, amino acids and herbs. Most often, the reason is that the ingredient in the plant (the property in the plant when found to be effective in healing) becomes listed as a Schedule F Drug by Health Canada.

In the name of public safety, NHPs are treated as Schedule F drugs and, therefore, manufacturers are required to apply for licensing. Also, some of these NHPs are now available only by prescription. Because of the number of pharmaceuticals that are marketed to doctors by major corporations, natural supplements and products are prescribed infrequently. Non-Canadian NHP manufacturers no longer even attempt to apply for licensing due to the costs involved. As stated by the NHPPA, "U.S. manufacturers put a self-imposed restriction on importing and selling NHPs in Canada because their makers cannot justify the expense, time, or effort that each NHP license application requires." When all is said and done, Canadian consumers have far fewer choices when it comes to buying NHPs. Furthermore, it's been reported that while these restrictions have not saved a single life, they have cost Canadian taxpayers more than $1 billion.

But the problems do not end there. As the NHFC suggests, many of the NHP regulations may be illegal:

(1) There is no act of Parliament that grants Health Canada the authority to regulate dietary supplements . . . it just doesn't exist. And (2), as has been pointed out so eloquently by Prime Minister Harper: Health is a provincial jurisdiction. Just because the Provinces are not addressing an area does not give Ottawa [the nation's capital] the legal right to fill it. And with zero deaths on record, dietary supplements do not meet the criteria to be dealt with at a federal criminal level.

It remains unclear who or what Health Canada is trying to protect through their strict regulations and bans. What is clear, however, is that Canadian citizens want better access to NHPs, even as the number of available products decreases with each passing year

Despite these setbacks, there have been some positive developments. In November 2011, the Canadian Health Food Association (CHFA), a nonprofit trade organization, publicly called upon Health Canada to develop and enact a new law governing natural health products, thereby exempting them from the jurisdiction of the Food and Drugs Act. A separate law for NHPs is attractive for several reasons: (1) It would properly define and correctly regulate NHPs; (2) it would avoid many of the drug requirements being applied to NHPs; (3) it would establish an appropriate safety model for NHPs that recognizes that supplements are intrinsically benign, that drugs are intrinsically dangerous, and that the relative safety of each is based on a completely different risk-benefit paradigm.

According to CHFA, a survey conducted by Ipsos-Reid clearly showed that "the public supports a new act for NHPs." More specifically, the survey found that seven in ten Canadians support a new law for NHP regulations. Carl Carter of the CHFA said that "the industry feels very strongly that full regulation is needed, but in the form of a new act, a Natural Health Products Act." Carter also stated that between 92 and 96 percent of CHFA members are behind the legislation; therefore, there is a "very strong mandate from [the CHFA] membership."

Still, there are some obstacles in the way of new legislation. Carter has pointed out, "One of the biggest obstacles we face is precisely the fact that . . . natural health products have such a great safety record." Ironically, it would be easier to make the case that existing regulations are insufficient if NHPs had a history of safety problems or adverse events. Furthermore, not all stakeholder groups support a new law for NHPs. As Gerry Harrington of Consumer Health Products Canada pointed out, "It would defy common sense to abandon [the NHP regulations] now and start over, when they've never really been enforced [thanks to NHP UPLAR provisions that allowed some products to remain on store shelves]."

In May 2012, the NHFC announced that it was going to protest Health Canada's bans and restrictions on NHPs by submitting a formal petition to the Canadian Supreme Court. According to a *Natural Products Insider* article from May 2012, "NHFC said it is concerned that the recent removal of more than 40,000 natural health products from the shelves in Canada have left consumers with no option but to purchase high-priced pharmaceutical drugs." If these endeavors are successful, the NHFC will obtain an injunction against Health Canada, inform the public about what is happening to NHPs, and launch a campaign against big pharmaceutical companies.

CONCLUSION

Although they may have been motivated by good intentions, it's clear that NHP regulations have thus far failed miserably. This should serve as a lesson to the U.S., which is in danger of going down the same path towards European-like supplement regulations. As things currently stand, it will be a long time before a less restrictive market for natural health products is restored in Canada. The final word, however, has not yet been spoken.

Conclusion

The FDA, Big Pharma, and the Future of Health Freedom

"They who can give up essential liberty to obtain a little temporary safety, deserve neither liberty nor safety."

—BENJAMIN FRANKLIN, 1775

This book began by looking at the various forces that spurred and shaped the natural health movement and its many manifestations in the United States. The public's growing interest in health in the nineteenth century was due in large part to anxieties created by social ills such as disease, food contamination, filthy cities, and deadly mainstream medicine—all of which were indirect results of the country's move towards industrialization.

Despite the steps that have been taken on a global scale to improve medicine, agriculture, food safety and purity, and access to supplements, some things still have not changed. Industry continues to threaten our health as well as our health freedom; only now the agencies and regulatory forces designed to protect us are part of the problem. The special interests that influence business and industry are the same ones that influence politicians and government authorities—the people who ultimately make the decisions that affect the environment, the quality of our food supply, the availability of supplements, and our ability to choose and afford natural treatments. The "marriage" of industry and decision-making bodies like the FDA has allowed special interests to supersede public interest and well-being. It has also allowed unfair restrictions on—and a lack of information about—potentially health-enhancing products. Meanwhile, the FDA and other agencies have continually turned a blind eye to true health dangers.

No case better reflects this than that of the pharmaceutical industry, whose power and influence over the FDA during the last several decades has greatly endangered public health. This issue is largely overlooked by the mainstream media, despite the fact that prescription drugs kill an estimated 100,000 Americans and injure an additional 2.2 million each year. Although a few pages on the history of the FDA's approval of unsafe drugs can hardly do the subject justice, it's important to highlight a few key examples of the agency's tainted record.

• **Troglitazone (Rezulin).** An anti-diabetic and anti-inflammatory drug developed by a Japanese pharmaceutical company, troglitazone was introduced in the U.S. by Parke-Davis, a subsidiary of Pfizer, in the late 1990s. The substance was reportedly linked to drug-induced hepatitis and liver toxicity, prompting an FDA medical officer to recommend non-approval. Nevertheless, troglitazone was approved by an FDA panel in January 1997. It wasn't withdrawn from the U.S. market until three years later, on March 22, 2000, after numerous reported cases of liver damage. According to attorney Jonathan Emord, author of 2008's *The Rise of Tyranny*, when all was said and done, the drug was implicated in 391 deaths, including 63 from liver failure.

• **Dexfenfluramine (Redux).** The lead FDA medical reviewer on this case, Dr. Leo Lutwak, told the *LA Times* in 2000 that he objected to the approval of this appetite suppressant in 1995, saying, "I, as the primary reviewer, felt the drug had low effectiveness and very high risk for neurotoxicity and pulmonary hypertension." Lutwak's immediate supervisor at the FDA, Dr. Solomon Sobel, also opposed market approval of dexfenfluramine, telling the *LA Times*, "I was supposed to sign off on that letter [approving Redux] . . . I told an [FDA manager] that I would *not* sign on it. If he wanted to approve it, *he* should sign it. And the record shows, *he's* the one who signed it." The drug was withdrawn from the U.S. market in September 1997 after a number of people taking the substance developed heart valve disease (aortic insufficiency), a condition characterized by the leaking of the aortic valve, which causes blood to flow in the opposite direction.

- **Rofecoxib (Vioxx).** A non-steroidal anti-inflammatory drug (NSAID) for osteoarthritis, rofecoxib was approved by the FDA on May 20, 1999, despite a pre-approval study indicating that those taking the drug had four times the risk of heart attack than patients who took naproxen, another anti-inflammatory medication. The FDA decided to accept the manufacturer's argument that this disparity was due to a cardio-protective effect of naproxen rather than a harmful effect of Vioxx, and the drug was approved.

Later, a randomized, placebo-controlled study found a higher rate of heart attack and other cardiovascular disorders among Vioxx users than patients who did not take any medication. Facing lawsuits, the manufacturer voluntarily withdrew Vioxx from the market in 2004. The damage had already been done, however, as the drug was connected to an estimated 28,000 cases of heart attack and sudden cardiac death. David Graham, a scientist for the FDA, later testified in front of Congress, stating that his supervisors pressured him to stay silent about the dangers of Vioxx and other drugs. He also pointed out the conflict of interest that exists when the office that monitors drug safety is controlled by the agency that approves the drugs in the first place.

- **Rosiglitazone (Avandia).** In April 1999, an FDA medical reviewer, Robert I. Misbin, reported to his supervisors that Avandia—a type 2 diabetes drug manufactured by GlaxoSmithKline (GSK)—appeared to increase the incidence of congestive heart failure. In an internal agency report dated April 2, 1999, Misbin warned that this concerns about the "deleterious long term effects on the heart should be addressed by requiring the manufacturer to provide adequate information in the label about changes in weight and lipids [blood fats]. A postmarketing study to address these issues needs to be a condition of approval." This recommendation was rejected, and on May 25, 1999, Avandia entered the U.S. market. In February 2006, another medical reviewer, Rosemary Johann-Liang, called for a black-box warning on Avandia's label to alert doctors and patients about the drug's cardiovascular risks. Her recommendation was also ignored.

Yet, science was not deterred. In May 2007, the *New England Journal of Medicine* published a critical review showing that Avandia increased the risk of heart attack by a staggering 43 percent. In June of the same year, during congressional hearings regarding the drug, former Congresswoman Diane Watson revealed that she had developed a heart murmur after taking Avandia and criticized the FDA commissioner for failing to include a warning on the label.

According to DrugWatch.com, serious cardiovascular side effects and potentially life-threatening complications from Avandia prompted tens of thousands of patients in the United States to file lawsuits against the drug's manufacturer, which could face up to $6 billion in liabilities. An FDA scientist quoted on the website stated that Avandia has been linked to as many as 100,000 heart attacks.

Although the FDA finally agreed to black-box warnings, Avandia was not removed from the market. According to Emord, "Pressured to keep the product on the market despite the heart risks, the [FDA drug advisory] committee produced a schizophrenic result." Although the committee agreed that Avandia increased cardiac risk in type 2 diabetics, it ultimately voted in favor of keeping the drug on the market.

• **Telithromycin (Ketek).** The first "ketolide" antibiotic to enter clinical use, telithromycin is used to treat mild to moderate community-acquired pneumonia. In February 2007, FDA medical reviewer David B. Ross testified to Congress that the FDA had approved the drug despite being aware that it could cause fatal liver damage, and that tens of millions of people would be exposed to it. Ross also stated that the FDA, ignoring objections from him and others, had knowingly allowed false information from a Ketek safety study to be presented to the drug advisory committee at a 2003 meeting to decide whether or not to approve telithromycin. Furthermore, Ross testified that the FDA had not told the committee that this falsified data was under criminal investigation.

Despite these serious concerns, Ketek was approved in April 2004. It remains on the market today, with more than 6.1 million prescriptions. Since its approval, the drug has been linked to dozens of cases of acute liver failure. According to Ross's testimony, the FDA responded by silencing internal criticism rather than removing the drug from the market.

• **SSRIs (Paxil, Zoloft, Effexor, and others).** In September 2003, an FDA medical reviewer discovered evidence that a class of antidepressant drugs, serotonin reuptake inhibitors (SSRIs), could increase the risk of suicidal thoughts in children. After the agency's initial attempts to suppress these findings, on September 14, 2004, the FDA advisory committee voted in favor of requiring SSRI manufacturers to include a black-box warning alerting users to the heightened risk of suicidal thoughts and tendencies. However, to date, no SSRIs have been removed from the market.

In addition to the cases already discussed, the FDA has been forced to remove or call for the withdrawal of a number of drugs from the market after they were linked to serious or fatal side effects. This list includes but is not limited to:

● Alosetron (Lotronex), a medication for irritable bowel syndrome reported to cause ischemic colitis.

● Cerivastatin (Baycol), a cholesterol-lowering drug that was said to cause severe muscle injury.

● Cisapride (Propulsid), a drug for night-time heartburn reported to cause heart arrhythmias and death.

● Temafloxacin (Omniflox), an antibiotic that was said to cause hemolytic anemia.

● Terfenadine (Seldane), an anti-histamine connected to heart arrhythmias and death.

● Trovafloxacin (Trovan), an antibiotic linked to acute liver failure and death.

● Valdecoxib (Bextra), a non-steroidal anti-inflammatory drug used to treat arthritis and painful menstruation that was connected to heart attack, stroke, and death.

In the 2011 book *Death by Medicine,* the authors point to a "very telling report" issued by the Government Accountability Office (GAO) stating that of the 198 drugs approved by the FDA between 1976 and 1985, 102 (51.5 percent) had "serious post-market risks." These risks included heart failure, stroke, anaphylaxis, kidney failure, liver failure, severe blood disorders, fetal toxicity, birth deformities, and blindness. Simply put, these medications were much more harmful than the conditions they were designed to treat.

As Jonathan Emord reported in his book, since the 1990s, there has been a steady stream of FDA scientists leaving the agency "when their consciences could no longer condone FDA approval of unsafe drugs." Almost without exception, each of these scientists has testified to Congress and the media that the FDA "owes" the drug industry, that the agency views the drug industry as a client, and that the FDA does the industry's bidding by approving drugs as safe when the evidence suggests otherwise. Emord wrote of the FDA's shameful history:

> [The agency's] record is one of silencing scientific criticism, eliminating evidence of dissent, hiding critical reviews of drugs from the public, inviting industry leaders to participate in internal management of the agency's medical reviewers, and coordinating with industry leaders to use public resources to defend the reputation of regulated firms. To say the FDA's Commissioners have gotten away with murder is to speak literally.

Offering further proof, Emord quotes Francesca Grifo, Senior Scientist and Director of the Scientific Integrity Program at the Union of Concerned Scientists, who said of the FDA, "Censoring scientists undermines our democracy and threatens public health. One stunning example: Vioxx. Fifty-five thousand Americans died because scientists at the Food and Drug Administration couldn't speak out."

There are few checks in place when it comes to keeping the FDA honest about drug safety. According to the authors of *Death by Medicine,* the Congressional Office of Technology Assessment (OTA), which existed from 1972 to 1995, was the U.S. government's "last honest agency," as it critically reviewed the state of the nation's healthcare system. But soon after the OTA issued a report detailing how financial interests control healthcare practice in the U.S., the OTA was disbanded by Congress.

The pharmaceutical industry's hold on the FDA is still very much a reality. This relationship has a central role in determining policies, regulations, and other decisions of the FDA Commissioner and other FDA officials, who may be (and have been) offered lucrative positions at drug companies, universities, and law and lobbying firms in return for their support. But unfortunately, its sphere of influence doesn't end with the FDA. In Jonathan Emord's words, the industry has created a "sophisticated, comprehensive, and unceasing program of influence peddling" that extends to medical professionals, institutions, and political heads—including the President.

With sales representatives numbering approximately 88,000, pharmaceutical companies regularly give gifts, free drug samples, and information promoting their drugs to doctors, teaching hospital staffs, and scientists who write for medical journals and respond to media inquiries. In addition, the industry influences medical research and literature via corporate sponsorship of clinical studies, symposia, medical journal supplements, and other widely circulated publications, as well as direct advertising. And through campaign contributions, gifts, lavish junkets, and the promise of industry-supported positions after leaving office, politicians also fall under the influence of drug companies. In his book, Emord eloquently explains this all-encompassing influence of the pharmaceutical industry in politics and beyond:

> The industry's success rate in blocking legislation against its interests and in securing passage of legislation in its favor is unparalleled. There is no other industry in the history of the United States, including the defense industry, that has enjoyed more largesse in the form of federal dollars transferred to them from the United States Treasury [for research and vaccines, for example] than the pharmaceutical industry. None has enjoyed more legal protection from competition than the pharmaceutical industry.

Meanwhile, information on the health benefits of supplements and natural medicine continues to be overlooked and suppressed; the food supply continues to be tainted with harmful chemical additives; the environment continues to suffer from unsustainable agricultural practices; and in countries like Canada, natural products are tightly controlled and even prohibited. Our right to be healthy, as well as our right to make choices about our health, is becoming increasingly compromised. Surely, the FDA is not the only factor at fault here. Nevertheless, a powerful case can be made that the agency has not always let public interest determine their decisions and inform their policies. And in the case of prescription drugs, the FDA willfully continues to put our health at risk.

But you can fight back and help win the struggle for health freedom. If everyone makes an effort to stay informed, become more politically active and engaged, and support the work of credible health-advocacy organizations, consumers will become a much more powerful force. By sending letters, signing petitions, and making donations when possible, you can help restore honesty to the FDA, as well as oppose Big Government skeptics who believe that Americans are incapable of making well-informed decisions when it comes to dietary supplements, natural health, and other forms of alternative medicine.

It is possible to take back our health and our health freedom if we take action. In the words of Jonathan Emord, "If that love of liberty that has inspired great Americans to sacrifice all to secure its blessings can be translated into political action in our day, we may yet see a restoration of the republic and a rekindling of liberty's sacred fire."

Bibliography

1. The Origins of the U.S. Natural Health Movement

Adams, Mark. *Mr. America: How Muscular Millionaire Bernarr Macfadden Transformed the Nation Through Sex, Salad, and the Ultimate Starvation Diet.* New York, NY: IT Books/HarperCollins, 2010.

Association of Physicians. *The Journal of Health.* [Reprints from the University of Michigan Library] 1829–1830.

Bartlett, Elisha. "On the Certainty of Medicine." *American Journal of Homeopathy.* Volume 3. 1849, p. 165.

Berman, Alex and Michael A. Flannery. *America's Botanico-Medical Movements: Vox Populi.* Binghamton, NY: Haworth Press, 2001.

Bobrow-Strain, Aaron. *White Bread: A Social History of the Store-Bought Loaf.* Boston, MA: Beacon Press, 2012.

Center for Food Safety. "Myths & Realities of GE Crops." The True Food Network. [Website] Retrieved from: http://truefoodnow.org/campaigns/genetically-engineered-foods/ge-crops/myths-realities-of-ge-crops/

City University of New York Graduate Center. "Cholera in 1849." Virtual New York [Website]. Retrieved from http://www.virtualny.cuny.edu/cholera/1849/cholera_1849_set.html

Dalton, JC. "Hydropathy." *The American Cyclopedia: A Popular Dictionary of General Knowledge*, vol. 9. George Ripley and Charles Dana, eds. New York: D. Appleton and Company, 1879.

Davoli, Elizabeth L. "Patent Medicines: Ethnic or Socioeconomic Indicators?" Presented at the First Annual South Central Historical Archeology Conference. Retrieved from: http://www.uark.edu/campus-resources/archinfo/SHACdavoli.pdf

Detmar, Bernhard. *Live Wisely—Live Well!* London, England: Thorsons, 1951.

Fee, Elizabeth. "Public Health and the State: The United States." *The History of Public Health and the Modern State.* Dorothy Porter, ed. New York, NY: Editions Rodopi, 1994.

Gormley, James J. "Coming of Age: The Evolution of the Natural Products Industry." *Health Products Business.* 49:4 (2003), pp. 16–22.

Kirchfeld, Friedhelm and Wade Boyle. *Nature Doctors: Pioneers in Naturopathic Medicine,* 2nd edition. Portland, OR: NCNM Press, 2005.

Graham, Sylvester. *Lectures on the Science of Human Life.* [Reprints from the University of Michigan Library] Battle Creek, MI: The Office of the Health Reformer, 1839.

Harmon, Kelly. *A Period of Deceit: The Patent Medicine Business Between 1865 and 1906.* [Bachelor's thesis] Asheville, NC: University of North Carolina at Asheville, 2003.

Hauser, Gayelord. *Look Younger, Live Longer.* Greenwich, CT: Fawcett Publications, 1950. Reprint, 1970.

Jackson, James C. *How to Treat the Sick Without Medicine.* New York, NY: Baker, Pratt & Co., 1870.

LaLanne, Jack. *Revitalize Your Life.* Winter Park, FL: Hastings House/Daytrips Publishers, 2003.

Maxwell, John. "The President's Message." *Health Foods Retailing.* 4:2 (1939), pp. 4.

McManis, Sam. "Raising the Bar: At 88, Fitness Guru Jack LaLanne Can Run Circles Around Those Half His Age." *San Francisco Chronicle.* January 19, 2003.

Medina, Miriam. "New York Tenement Life." The History Box. [Website] Retrieved from: http://www.thehistorybox.com/ny_city/tenement_life_ gallery.htm

Mitchell, Dennis. "George Barker Windship, MD." United States All-Around Weightlifting Association. March 2, 2010. Retrieved from: http://www.usawa.com/george-barker-windship-md/

Murray, Frank. *More Than One Slingshot: How the Health Food Industry is Changing America.* Richmond, VA: Marlborough House, 1984.

Numbers, Ronald L. *Prophetess of Health: A Study of Ellen G. White,* 3rd edition. Grand Rapids, MI: William B. Eerdmans Publishing Company, 2008.

Redman, Nina E. *Food Safety: A Reference Handbook,* 2nd edition. Santa Barbara, CA: ABC-CLIO, 2007.

Sappol, Michael, ed. *Hidden Treasure: The National Library of Medicine.* New York, NY: Blast Books, 2012.

Sinclair, Upton. *The Jungle.* New York: Doubleday, 1906.

Swerdlow, Joel L. *Nature's Medicine: Plants That Heal.* Washington, DC: National Geographic Society, 2000.

Todd, Jan. "'Strength Is Health': George Barker Windship and the First American Weight Training Boom." *Iron Game History.* September 1993. Retrieved from: http://www.la84foundation.org/SportsLibrary/IGH/ IGH0301/IGH0301c.pdf

Weider, Joe and Ben Weider. *Brothers of Iron.* Champaign, IL: Sports Publishing LLC, 2006.

White, Ellen G. *Ministry of Healing.* Nampa, ID: Pacific Press, 1909.

Whorton, James C. "The History of Complementary and Alternative Medicine." *Essentials of Complementary and Alternative Medicine.* Wayne B. Jonas and Jeffrey S. Levin, eds. Baltimore, MD: Lippincott Williams & Wilkins, 1999.

Yagoda, Ben. "The True Story of Bernard Macfadden: Lives and Loves of the Father of the Confession Magazine." *American Heritage.* 33(1): 1981. Retrieved from: http://www.americanheritage.com/content/true-story-bernard-macfadden

2. Harvest of Shame: Business, Politics, and the Food Supply

American Farmland Trust. "American Farmland Trust Urges Congress to Consider Environmental and Conservation Impacts of New Farm Bill; Calls for Conservation Compliance for Crop Insurance Eligibility." [Press release] March 15, 2012. Retrieved from: http://www.farmland.org/news/pressreleases/2012/Consider-the-Environmental-Impacts-of-Farm-Safety-Net-Reform.asp

Biodynamic Farming and Gardening Association. "What is Biodynamics?" [Webpage] 2012. Retrieved from: https://www.biodynamics.com/biodynamics.html

Center for Food Safety. "New Report Reveals Dramatic Rise in Pesticide Use on Genetically Engineered (GE) Crops Due to the Spread of Resistant Weeds." The True Food Network. [Website] November 17, 2009. Retrieved from: http://true-foodnow.org/2009/11/17/new-report-reveals-dramatic-rise-in-pesticide-use-on-genetically-engineered-ge-crops-due-to-the-spread-of-resistant-weeds/

Cornell University Department of Horticulture. "Ecogardening Factsheet #9." 1993. Retrieved from: http://www.gardening.cornell.edu/factsheets/ecogardening/imp-soilcov.html

Engdahl, F. W. "Monsanto Buys 'Terminator' Seeds Company." Center for Research on Globalization. August 27, 2006. Retrieved from: http://www.globalresearch.ca/monsanto-buys-terminator-seeds-company/3082

Environmental Protection Agency. "The Quality of Our Nation's Waters: A Summary of the National Water Quality Inventory: 1998 Report to Congress." Washington, DC: Office of Water, June 2000. Retrieved from: http://water.epa.gov/lawsregs/guidance/cwa/305b/upload/2000_07_07_305b_98report_98brochure.pdf

——. "What You Should Know About Pfiesteria piscicida." Washington, DC: Office of Wetlands, Oceans, and Watersheds, January 1998.

Gormley, James J. "The Organic Movement: Protecting Our Food." *Better Nutrition* 59:4 (April 1997), pp. 8.

Grace Communications Foundation. "Soil Quality." [Webpage] Retrieved from: http://www.gracelinks.org/207/soil-quality

Hoppe, Robert A. and David E. Banker. "Structure and Finances of U.S. Farms: Family Farm Report, 2010 Edition." USDA Economic Research Service. July 2010. Retrieved from: http://www.ers.usda.gov/media/184479/eib66_1_.pdf

Johns Hopkins Bloomberg School of Public Health. "Teaching the Food System." Retrieved from: http://www.jhsph.edu/research/centers-and-institutes/teaching-the-food-system/curriculum/history_of_food.html

Leverton, Ruth M. "Nutrition in Perspective." Proceedings of the USDA National Nutrition Education Conference. November 2–4, 1971.

Mann, Charles C. "Our Good Earth." *National Geographic.* September 2008, pp. 80–106.

Marks, Robbin. "Cesspools of Shame: How Factory Farm Lagoons and Sprayfields Threaten Environmental and Public Health." National Resources Defense Council and the Clean Water Network, 2001. Retrieved from: http://www.nrdc.org/water/pollution/cesspools/cesspools.pdf

Minnesota Department of Agriculture. "Back by popular demand—the Minnesota Grown Directory!" [Press release] May 7, 2012. Retrieved from: http://www.mda.state.mn.us/news/releases/2012/nr-2012-05-07-mngrow.aspx

——."Energy and Sustainable Agriculture." 2012. Retrieved from: https://www.mda.state.mn.us/en/about/divisions/amd/esap.aspx

Morgan, Dan, et al. "How to Spend an Extra $15 Billion." *Washington Post.* July—December 2006. Retrieved from: http://www.washingtonpost.com/wp-srv/nation/interactives/farmaid/

Ohio State University Department of Horticulture and Crop Science. "Fact Sheet: Cover Crop Fundamentals." Retrieved from: http://ohioline.osu.edu/agf-fact/0142.html

Oldways Preservation Trust. "Founder & History." [Webpage] Retrieved from: http://oldwayspt.org/about-us/founder-history

Pimentel, David, et al. "Environmental and Economic Costs of Soil Erosion and Conservation Benefits." *Science* 267:5201 (1995), pp. 1117–1123.

Robbins, John. *Diet for a New America.* Peterborough, NH: Stillpoint Publishers, 1987.

——. *The Food Revolution.* Berkley, CA: Conari Press, 2001.

Roosevelt, Franklin D. "Letter from President to all State Governors on a Uniform Soil Conservation Law." February 26, 1937. *The American Presidency Project.* [Website] Gerhard Peters and John T. Woolley, eds. http://www.presidency.ucsb.edu/ws/?pid=15373

Sciamacco, Sara. "Top 10 Things You Should Know About The Farm Bill." The Environmental Working Group. June 27, 2011. Retrieved from: http://www.ewg.org/agmag/2011/06/top-10-things-you-should-know-about-the-farm-bill/

Shiva, Vandana. *Stolen Harvest: The Hijacking of the Global Food Supply.* Cambridge, MA: South End Press, 2000.

Slow Food USA. "Good, Clean and Fair." 2010. Retrieved from: http://www.slowfoodusa.org/index.php/slow_food/good_clean_fair/2010

Soroptimist International. "Food Systems Facing Climate Change—Creating Impact." December 11, 2012. Retrieved from: http://www.soroptimistinternational.org/who-we-are/news/post/401-food-systems-facing-climate-change-creating-impact

Visser, Ben, et al. "Potential Impacts of Genetic Use Restriction Technologies (GURTs) on Agrobiodiversity and Agricultural Production Systems." Background Study Paper No. 15. Retrieved from: ftp://ftp.fao.org/docrep/fao/meeting/015/aj627e.pdf

3. Politics, the FDA, and Your Health Choices: The Great Health Freedom Battles in U.S. History

Aarts, Thomas. "DSHEA Ten Years Later: How Did We Get Here?" *Natural Foods Merchandiser* 25:3 (March 1, 2004), pp. 38. Retrieved from: http://newhope360.com/dshea-10-years-later-how-did-we-get-here-0

Anderson, Mark. "Dr. Royal Lee." [Website] Retrieved from: www.drroyalee.com

Citizens for Health. "The FDA Goes Back to the Drawing Board on NDI Draft Guidance!" June 20, 2011. Retrieved from: http://www.citizens.org/the-fda-goes-back-to-drawing-board-on-ndi-draft-guidance/

Food and Drug Administration. "Harvey W. Wiley: Pioneer Consumer Activist." *FDA Consumer.* January—February 2006. Retrieved from: http://www.fda.gov/AboutFDA/WhatWeDo/History/CentennialofFDA/HarveyW.Wiley/default.htm

Huberman, Mark A. "My Dad: A Great Hygienist." National Health Association. January 15, 2009. Retrieved from: http://tinyurl.com/nha-max-huberman

Lee, Royal. "The Battlefront for Better Nutrition." *The Interpreter.* July 15, 1950. Retrieved from: https://seleneriverpress.com/archive-articles/163-lee-the-battlefront-for-better-nutrition

Lutz, Karl B. "Protest Against Persecution of the Health Movement by the Food and

Drug Administration." Monrovia, CA: National Health Federation, 1963. Retrieved from: http://tinyurl.com/karl-lutz-nhf

McBean, Eleanor. *The Poisoned Needle*. Pomeroy, WA: Health Research Books, 1957.

Miller, Clinton Ray. Testimony to the House of Representatives Subcommittee on Public Health and Environment of the Committee on Interstate and Foreign Commerce. Hearing, October 29–31, 1973. Serial No. 93-58. Stock No. 5270-02217. Washington, DC: U.S. Government Printing Office, 1974.

Morris, David. "Royal Lee, DDS: Father of Natural Vitamins." Western A. Price Foundation. January 1, 2000. Retrieved from: http://www.westonaprice.org/nutrition-greats/royal-lee

Passwater, Richard. "FDA Injustices Against the Health Food Industry." *Whole Foods Magazine*. August 2005. Retrieved from: http://www.drpasswater.com/nutrition_library/Nov_05/Murray_FDA_Struggle_final.html

Reinhardt, Claudia and Bill Ganzel. "1930s Farm Life." Wessels Living History Farm. [Website] 2003. Retrieved from: http://www.livinghistoryfarm.org/farminginthe30s/life_01.html

Wiley, Harvey W. *The History of a Crime Against the Food Law*. Washington, DC: 1929.

Williams, Elizabeth and Stephanie Carter. *The A-Z Encyclopedia of Food Controversies and the Law*. Santa Barbara, CA: Greenwood/ABC-CLIO, 2010.

4. The Global Fix: Food Insecurity, Supplement Regulation, and Codex

Alliance for Natural Health. "Codex—Government and Corporate Control of Our Food Supply." 2010. Retrieved from: http://www.anhcampaign.org/campaigns/codex

Bock, Alan. "The Vitamin Police." *The Orange County Register*. August 15, 2005. Retrieved from: http://www.lewrockwell.com/ocregister/vitamin-police.html

Blythman, Joanna. "Health Supplements: R.I.P." *The Guardian*. September 13, 2002. Retrieved from: http://www.guardian.co.uk/society/2002/sep/14/medicineandhealth.lifeandhealth

Codex Alimentarius Commission. "Guidelines for Vitamin and Mineral Food Supplements." CAC/GL 55, 2005.

——. "Official Report of the Codex Alimentarius Commission, 28th Session." FAO/WHO. FAO Headquarters, Rome, Italy. July 4–9, 2005.

Denton, Sally. *The Plots Against the President*. New York: Bloomsbury Press, 2012.

Joint FAO/WHO Food Standards Programme. *Understanding the Codex Alimentarius*, 3rd edition. Rome: World Health Organization/ Food and Agriculture Organization of the United Nations, 2006. Retrieved from: ftp://ftp.fao.org/codex/ Publications/understanding/Understanding_EN.pdf

Gardner, Gary and Brian Halweil. *Underfed and Overfed: The Global Epidemic of Malnutrition.* Washington, DC: Worldwatch Institute, 2000.

Lupien, J. R. "The Codex Alimentarius Commission: International Science-Based Standards, Guidelines, and Recommendations." *AgBioForum* 3:4 (2000), pp. 192–196.

Randell, Alan. "Codex Alimentarius: How It All Began." FAO Corporate Document Repository, 1995. Retrieved from: http://www.fao.org/docrep/v7700t/v7700t09.htm

Shaw, D. John. *World Food Security: A History Since 1945.* Hampshire, England: Palgrave Macmillan, 2007.

Shepherd, Rose. "Nil By Mouth." *The Observer.* February 28, 2004. Retrieved from: http://www.guardian.co.uk/society/2004/feb/29/health.shopping

Smith, Jean Edward. *FDR.* New York, NY: Random House, 2008.

Turner, James. "Codex Alert on Dietary Supplements." The Weston A. Price Foundation. August 3, 2005. Retrieved from: http://tinyurl.com/jim-turner-codex-alert

——. "Update on Codex Alimentarius." The Weston A. Price Foundation. October 30, 2009. Retrieved from: http://tinyurl.com/jim-turner-codex-update

United Nations. "UN Commission Adopts Safety Guidelines for Vitamin and Food Supplements." UN News Centre. July 11, 2005. Retrieved from: http://tinyurl.com/codex-adopts-guidelines

Wood, Curtis, Jr. *Overfed but Undernourished.* New York, NY: Tower Publications, 1971.

World Trade Organization. "Agreement on the Application of Sanitary and Phytosanitary Measures." April, 1994. Retrieved from: http//www.wto.org/english/docs_e/legal_e/15sps_01_e.htm

5. The Canada Example

"Advocacy Group Vows to Fight Health Canada." *Natural Products Insider.* May 29, 2012. Retrieved from: http://www.naturalproductsinsider.com/news/2012/05/advocacy-group-vows-to-fight-health-canada.aspx

Caisse, Rene. "The First Treatments." *Bracebridge Examiner.* January 1979. Retrieved from: http://www.essiacinfo.org/caisse_pop_2.htm

Consumer Health Products Canada. "Natural Health Product Regulations: Common Sense Dictates that They Should Not Be Abandoned Without Ever Having Been Fully Enforced." [Press Release] November 17, 2011. Retrieved from: http://www.chpcanada.ca/index.cfm?fuseaction=main.dspFile&FileID=207

First Nations Health Council. "FNHC Welcomes New Suicide and Self-Harm Child and Youth Report Recommendations." [News release] November 16, 2012.

Retrieved from: http://www.fnhc.ca/index.php/news/article/fnhc_welcomes_ new_suicide_and_self_harm_child_and_youth_report_recommendati/

Glum, Gary. *Calling of an Angel.* Los Angeles, CA: Silent Walker Publishing, 1998.

Gormley, James J. "CHFA Calls for a New Law for Natural Health Products." *Nutritional Outlook.* April 13, 2012. Retrieved from: http://www.nutritionaloutlook.com/ article/canadian-nhp-regulations-5-9656

Harrison, John R. *International Regulation of Natural Health Products.* Boca Raton, FL: Universal Publishers, 2008.

Health Canada. "ICH [International Conference on Harmonisation]." Retrieved from: http://www.hc-sc.gc.ca/dhp-mps/prodpharma/applic-demande/guide-ld/ ich/index-eng.php

Leacock, Stephen. *The Mariner of St. Malo: A Chronicle of the Voyages of Jacques Cartier.* Toronto, 1915; Project Gutenberg, 2001. Retrieved from: http://www.gutenberg.org/files/4077/4077-h/4077-h.htm

Lloyd, Iva. *The History of Naturopathic Medicine: A Canadian Perspective.* Toronto, Canada: McArthur and Co., 2009.

Natural Health Product Protection Association "The Charter of Health Freedom." 2008. Retrieved from: http://www.charterofhealthfreedom.org/images/stories/ docs/charterofhealthfreedom.pdf

——. "Health Canada's Tactics: Losing NHPs Over Safety Or Corporate Profits?" Retrieved from: http://www.charterofhealthfreedom.org/index.php?/health-canadas-tactics

——. "Health Freedom Timeline: Cutting a Long Story Short." 2009. Retrieved from: http://www.charterofhealthfreedom.org/index.php?/health-control-timeline

Nelson, Marilyn. "Letter to Leona Aglukkaq." National Health Freedom Canada. March 19, 2012. Retrieved from: http://naturalhealthfreedomcanada.com/wp-content/uploads/2012/03/Sworn-Affidavit-20-March-2012.pdf

Obomsawin, Raymond. "Traditional Medicine for Canada's First Peoples." March 2007. Retrieved from: http://www.soilandhealth.org/02/0203cat/020337.traditional.medicine.pdf

"Spotlight: Essiac (René Caisse's Herbal Remedy)." [Webpage] Campaign for Truth in Medicine. Retrieved from: http://www.campaignfortruth.com/Eclub/170310/ CTM-essiac.htm

Starling, Shane. "Canadian Health Products Bill Draws Criticism." *Nutraingredients-USA.com.* May 16, 2008. Retrieved from: http://www.nutraingredients-usa.com/Regulation/Canadian-health-products-bill-draws-criticism

About the Author

James J. Gormley is an award-winning health journalist, medical editor, and author. As Editor-in-Chief of *Better Nutrition* from 1995 to 2002, he helped change the landscape of natural health reporting in the United States by pioneering science-centered coverage. Later, he served as the Editorial Director of the *Vitamin Retailer* magazine group, where he focused on shedding light on supplement misinformation.

Between 2002 and 2006, James managed regulatory and scientific affairs for Nutrition 21, where he played a key role in securing international market approval for high-quality supplement ingredients. He also attended the Oldways Conference on cross-cultural food issues as a U.S. delegate in 2001, as well as Codex Alimentarius Commission meetings in Paris and Rome in 2005.

James has been an unflagging crusader for both consumers and the responsible core of the supplement industry, and has always sought to unite the two constituencies. Currently, he is the Senior Policy Advisor and Vice President of Citizens for Health, and a member of the Scientific Advisory Board for the Natural Health Research Institute. He also writes for *Nutritional Outlook* magazine, SupplySide Community, and his own health politics blog, "The Gormley Files," and is the author of five books, including *The User's Guide to Brain-Boosting Supplements*.

Index

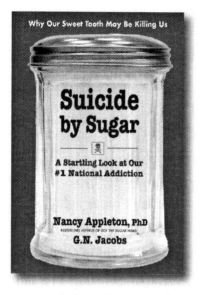

Why Our Sweet Tooth May Be Killing Us

Suicide by Sugar

A Startling Look at Our
#1 National Addiction

Nancy Appleton, PhD

G.N. Jacobs

SUICIDE BY SUGAR

A Startling Look at Our #1 National Addiction

Nancy Appleton, PhD, and G.N. Jacobs

It is a dangerous addictive white powder that can be found in abundance throughout this country. It is not illegal. In fact, it is available in or near playgrounds, schools, workplaces, homes, and vacation spots. It is in practically everything we eat and drink, and, once we're hooked on it, the cravings can be overwhelming. This white substance of abuse is sugar. Once associated only with cavities and simple weight gain, it is now linked to a host of devastating health conditions including cancer, epilepsy, dementia, hypoglycemia, obesity, and more. In this book, sugar addiction expert Dr. Nancy Appleton and health writer G.N. Jacobs not only expose the exorbitant levels of sugar we ingest, but also document the connection between our current health crisis and our sweet tooth.

Suicide by Sugar begins with the story of Dr. Appleton's battle with her own sugar addiction. Next, the authors examine all the frightening (and little known) things that can go wrong when people consume too much sugar—from increased susceptibility to disease to imbalanced body chemistry. The authors go on to discuss the various ways scientists measure sugar's impact on blood glucose, and explain why these statistics cannot be solely relied on when choosing foods. They provide shocking information about the amount of sugar found in many popular foods and beverages, and an in-depth discussion of the ailments now associated with excessive sugar consumption. Finally, Dr. Appleton's easy-to-follow, effective lifestyle plan—complete with recipes—guides you in eliminating sugar from your life.

$15.95 US • 192 pages • 6 x 9-inch quality paperback • ISBN 978-0-7570-0306-6

KILLER COLAS

The Hard Truth About Soft Drinks

Nancy Appleton, PhD, and G.N. Jacobs

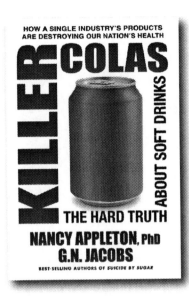

It's as American as fast food, ice cream, and apple pie. So why are people saying all those nasty things about soda? The answer is simple: Those nasty things are all true. While the facts may be hard to swallow, it is high time we address the damage being done to our well-being due to our long-running love affair with soft drinks and other sweetened beverages. In *Killer Colas,* Dr. Nancy Appleton and G.N. Jacobs provide a startling picture of an industry hell-bent on making a hefty profit at the ultimate expense of the country's health.

Over the last few decades, the sale of soft drinks, energy beverages, sports drinks, and enhanced waters has exploded, as has the incidence of obesity, diabetes, hypertension, heart disease, cancer, and stroke. *Killer Colas* looks at the origin of this downward spiral. The book traces the history and staggering growth of the soft drink industry, explores the powerful influence it has achieved through media-savvy advertising and marketing techniques, and examines the many harmful ingredients that these companies include in their most prized and popular formulas. In addition, it offers evidence of the frighteningly addictive properties of soft drinks, as well as research that links America's consumption of sweetened beverages to its overall decline in health.

In light of the country's overwhelming health crisis, the consequences of drinking soda and other sweetened beverages can no longer be ignored. *Killer Colas* exposes the facts behind a habit that is just as dangerous and destructive as smoking. Moreover, it suggests concrete solutions to this widespread problem, giving hope to a nation desperately in need of a healthful way forward. Once you have read this book, you will never look at soft drinks in the same way again.

$15.95 US • 144 pages • 6 x 9-inch quality paperback • ISBN 978-0-7570-0341-7

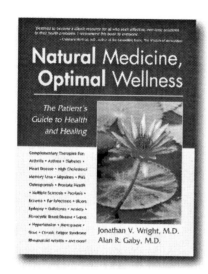